LOVE
PRESCRIPTION

LOVE PRESCRIPTION

*Ending the War Between
Black Men and Women*

JEFFREY GARDERE, PH.D.

Dafina
BOOKS

KENSINGTON PUBLISHING CORP.
http://www.kensingtonbooks.com

DAFINA BOOKS are published by

Kensington Publishing Corp.
850 Third Avenue
New York, NY 10022

All Kensington titles, imprints, and distributed lines are available at special quantity discounts for bulk purchases for sales promotion, premiums, fund-raising, educational or institutional use.

Special book excerpts or customized printings can also be created to fit specific needs. For details, write or phone the office of the Kensington Special Sales Manager: Kensington Publishing Corp., 850 Third Avenue, New York, NY 10022, Attn: Special Sales Department. Phone: 1-800-221-2647.

Dafina Books and the Dafina logo Reg. U.S. Pat. & TM Off.

Library of Congress Card Catalogue Number: 2002102155

ISBN 0-7582-0251-2

First Printing: December 2002
10 9 8 7 6 5 4 3 2 1

Printed in the United States of America

To my children, Q'vanaa Elektra, Puma-Xavier,
Sebastian Oskar, Baby X (in utero)
and their mom, Deyanira.
I love you all very much!

Acknowledgments

First and foremost, I offer my gratitude and appreciation to my co-writer, collaborator and soul sister, Dr. Elena Oumano. Not only did she help me put into words the psychological process behind dysfunctional relationships, but she was also instrumental with creating many of the healing prescriptions. It is her writing skills, expertise in human relationships, and creativity that has breathed life into this book.

Many thanks to Barbara Lowenstein, who has been both agent and mom. Barbara has not only taught me how to create innovative book projects, but also how to promote them. I feel very privileged to be among her stable of writers.

Karen Thomas has been not only a great editor but a good sport in allowing me to provide advice the "Dr. Jeff" way. I look forward to a long history with Karen and Dafina Books.

A special thanks to my good friend Karen Taylor for her encouragement and support. Also to Gary Pauyo, who ran my companies while I was swamped with writing.

Last and not least I am extremely grateful to all the patients, friends, brothers and sisters, who have fought in and peacefully ended the war between black men and women.

CONTENTS

LOVE
PRESCRIPTION

INTRODUCTION

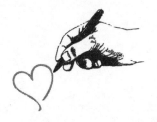

BULLETIN FROM THE FRONT LINES

If this is the love the old folks told me about
Man, I'm in trouble,
I'm in real big trouble.
Someone please call 911
                    —Wyclef Jean, "911"

Everyone knows about the war on terrorism, but few realize that another war is raging right here at home. You won't see the battle footage on CNN, but that doesn't make this conflict any less fierce. The combatants? Black men vs. black women. Compared to the schoolyard scuffles between their white, Hispanic, and Asian counterparts, the battle between black men and women seems like another world war.

I'm clinical psychologist Dr. Jeff Gardere, a.k.a. Dr. Jeff, and I monitor the war every day from my four psychotherapy clinics. I work primarily with black singles and couples, the walking wounded who provide me with regular updates from their personal battlegrounds.

I also keep up with current war developments as a radio talk show host and guest expert on national radio and television talk shows, such as *Ricki Lake, Montel Williams, Court TV,* and *Sally Jesse Raphael*, where I offer closing observations on the theater of dysfunctional relationships that has just played out on your television screen.

I try to keep it real at all times, no holds barred. This war is too serious not to report the absolute truth.

Let me begin by describing what happened one morning on *Hit It*, a popular NYC–based radio show I hosted for nearly two years. A woman named Chevelle called in the midst of a heated discussion about how far some sisters will go to find "love." The board engineer signaled a call waiting on line three, and I greeted the caller in my usual hype style:

"Good morning; let's hit it!"

"Dr. Jeff? Hi, this is Chevelle, from the Bronx. Dr. Jeff, I'm in big trouble and I really need your help," a woman said in a breathless rush.

"Whatever it is, don't worry. We can work it out," I assured her.

"I don't know if you can help me," Chevelle replied. "Let me tell you what's happened. I met this really nice guy, and we had a vibe. He had a good job as a licensed plumber, he drove a flashy red vintage BMW, he had nice manners, and he was fabulous in bed."

"So, what's the problem?" I asked.

"Dr. Jeff, do you believe he waited until after we'd done the nasty to tell me that he'd been married for fifteen years and had three kids?"

Nothing new there.

"So you dropped him like a bad habit, right?" I asked, though I was sure she hadn't.

"Well, not exactly," Chevelle admitted. "We're still involved."

"Why are you still involved, when *I* know that *you* know there's no future with a married man?" I didn't wait for her answer before asking another question: "How old are you?"

"I'm thirty-one, Dr. Jeff," Chevelle snapped, as if her "advanced" age were justification for dallying with a married man.

"You know, it's not too late to get out of this mess," I told her. "You can't be proud of this relationship. You should be enjoying yourself right now instead of being miserable. Despite what you may think, this is your youth right now, the time to make yourself available to the good single black men out there. And they are out there, believe me."

"Well, it's even more complicated than that," Chevelle finally admitted. "I don't mind giving him up, but there's a bigger problem." She paused.

I just knew she was about to come up with something really deep, but for her sake I hoped she wasn't going to say she was pregnant.

She clearly wanted me to say it for her, so I did.

"Don't tell me, you 'did it,'" I said. She knew what I meant.

"I did it,'" Chevelle admitted. "I'm three months pregnant for him."

"What future do you have with this married man?" I asked again.

"Well, I'm waiting for him to leave his wife and help me raise our child," Chevelle replied somewhat sheepishly.

"What makes you think he's going to do that?" I asked. "Has he promised that he'll leave his wife for you?"

"Not exactly," Chevelle answered. "That's why I called you, because I'm getting nervous. I haven't heard from him for two weeks."

Whether she realized it or not, this young lady had called for help, not so I could support her fantasies about this man and the family they were going to enjoy together. Somewhere deep down inside, she was reaching out for a reality check. So I laid it out for her. I said that she should not count on this man to leave his wife and children and help her raise their child. A married man's promise isn't worth the paper it's not written on. I believe in a woman's right to choose, so I asked how she felt about having an abortion. "This might be my only chance to have a child," Chevelle said. She wanted this baby, and according to her religion, abortion is a sin.

Chevelle was beginning to wake up to reality, and I wanted to leave her with a solid understanding of her options.

I told her what I would tell any other woman in a similar situation. The problem wasn't just this married man or even the pregnancy. It's easy to point the finger at the bow wow brother, but the real problem was Chevelle. She needed to take a look within to figure out why she had allowed herself to get into this chaotic, stressful, and even dangerous situation. Was it because she believed this was the best she could do and/or all she deserved? If a woman gets pregnant by a married man or any man who is not committed to her, she has to realize that she will raise this child on her own. She needs to take a long, hard look at her emotional baggage. Her self-esteem has to be at rock bottom if she's willing to settle for someone who doesn't love her or for another woman's leftovers.

Women who settle, neglect to take that long, hard look within, and that's why they usually find themselves jumping into the same dead-end situations over and over. Inevitably, they wind up feeling used, abused, and confused.

Black women like Chevelle usually defend their destructive relationships or relationship patterns by claiming they have no other choice. That when it comes to good single black men, the pickings are slim to none. That's why they're "forced" to settle for no-good men and unhealthy relationships.

Now, I've been a single black man, and, like most unattached brothers, I got my groove on every chance I got, with as many women as possible. I was young; I had a Ph.D., and I lived in New

York City. Believe me, it was easy. Today, I'm a husband and father to our three children. I've moved from being an enthusiastic player of war games to a state of peaceful surrender. I wrote this book to spread my gospel of peace to all my brothers and sisters.

"I know what it's like out there," I told Chevelle. "I know it's tough for a good woman looking for a good man. Brothers are running games, no doubt. But the real problem is that sisters keep falling for the 'same ol' okey doke,' then getting angrier and angrier at each disappointment and betrayal. Every man knows he can throw out the most tired lyric, and the law of averages will still work in his favor. I'm talking about single men, married men, blue-collar men, professional men—all shapes, sizes, and kinds of men. Sooner or later, some female will take the bait. But falling for a line is like hypnosis: You can only be put under if you are willing to go there."

I want to tell all the other sisters out there what I told Chevelle: You've got the power. You can refuse whatever situations aren't good for you and choose to pursue what you really want. The real problem is that most of you don't even recognize that you have that power of choice. You allow yourself to be victimized by the misguided notion that "no good black men are out there, so I might as well settle for whatever I can get." That's just the excuse you give yourself whenever you get lonely and give up by impetuously settling for familiar yet negative situations. That excuse keeps you stuck and screwed, and that's why you're so angry right now. Chevelle was so furious with this married man—as you may be furious with the men who've let you down—that she was ready to tar all brothers with the same brush. Not all brothers are dogs. It's on you, my sisters, to hold out for the good ones.

The next day on my radio show, my listeners and I tackled another hot-button subject: infidelity in marriage. The engineer signaled a call on line two. Lo and behold, it was a married sister named Joanie.

"Let's hit it, baby," I greeted her.

"Dr. Jeff, 'member that woman Chevelle who was telling you about that married man?" she asked in a melodic Jamaican lilt. "Well, Dr. Jeff, I hope you're sitting down right now, because that's *my* married man, *my* husband, the father of *our* three children. That's *my* red BMW, and I'm the one who set him up in his plumbing business."

I was speechless. I really didn't know what to say, but I can tell you what I was thinking: "This is great radio, but at the expense of yet another black relationship."

"Are you sure?" I ventured.

"Yes, I'm sure," she retorted, rage suddenly turned up full blast. "Plus, a lot of my girlfriends, and God knows who else, heard your show yesterday. I've been humiliated before my friends and the world! I'm ready to kill him for doing this to me!"

"Have you confronted him?" I asked timidly.

"I sure as hell did," she retorted, "and his sorry behind is already gone! I threw his clothes out the window and him out the door! And I'm never letting that dog back in!"

"You're not at all willing to talk this over with him, to see if things can be worked out?" I suggested gamely.

"My dear," she drawled lethally. "The only subject he and I can discuss is D-I-V-O-R-C-E and how soon he's returning my red Beemer. And by the way, I owe you, Dr. Jeff. I'll be using the tape

I recorded of Chevelle telling all on the radio for my divorce proceedings."

The wife dropped the bomb, and Chevelle dropped the plumber. This sad tale ended with three people miserable and two homes without a dad.

Similar scenarios of distrust, faithlessness, resentment, and bitterness play out between countless other black men and women every day. This war is no joke. When it comes to love and marriage, today's brothers and sisters are in trouble—real big trouble!

Studies show that the current divorce rate for blacks is four times greater than it was in 1960 and double that of the general population. Black men and black women are locked in an intense struggle, and the battles grow fiercer by the day. Each side distrusts the other deeply, dislikes each other intensely, and unless they find ways to overcome these issues so they can make genuine and lasting love connections, the war will never end.

Whose side am I on in this ongoing conflict? Everyone's, because we're all losers in this war.

I do admit to a lifelong weakness for the underdog, and that's one reason why I'm prepared to give it up to the sisters. That's right, this book provides sisters with the complete 411, straight from the male opposition's war room, because when it comes to the ravages of this war, let's be honest: sisters suffer more.

Out there in the cold, hard world of single 'n' mingle, black women seriously outnumber black men. The dating world is the brother's oyster. You know what I'm talking about. Every evening, crowds of women floss for half as many brothers in packed after-work bars and nightclubs. Every Sunday, at church socials, it's the same scenario. As Chris Rock observes, "A man is as faithful as his options." And we've got plenty of those. I've seen it over and over:

smart, interesting women go without, while nerdy, Erkel-looking brothers get play galore from the ladies.

We brothers *believe* we have the choices, call the shots, and don't agonize like the sisters over the hardships involved in trying to form a quality relationship.

Actually, few black men believe they are hurting at all, though a series of failed relationships can leave a brother as romantically dissatisfied and emotionally disabled as a sister. Black men are in pain; they're just in denial about their pain. Leave it up to us, and we'd procreate with as many women as possible, as if sex were the panacea for all our emotional problems. We blindly hunt that make-me-feel-ever-so-right sex, but that's not the real answer.

Brothers, you may believe polishing your game is the way to win the war and achieve happiness. I'm going to show you the error of your ways. This book will prove that you need to drop the strategies and defenses so we can create new, win-win romantic situations in which everyone's happy.

That dream is the reason why I'm telling the truth about black love—or the lack of it—from every angle of the black man's and woman's points of view. I remember during the first months when *Hit It* came on the air. Brothers burned up the phone lines: "Yo! Dr. Jeff! I mean, wassup? Why you telling the females all our secrets!"

I wouldn't reveal our secrets if I didn't hold out hope for us. I may seem at times to address the ladies, but the knowledge I impart here is just as valuable to men. I'm prepared for the haters among you, and I want you to know that I'm giving up the playbook for the black man's own good. I'm giving up the truth about the black man's and black woman's romantic antics, because once sisters and brothers have new, more accurate insights into how the other side thinks and behaves, we'll all have a better shot at working it out.

Sisters, when you finish highlighting the good parts, pass this book on to a needy brother. Brothers, don't be afraid of this book. In fact, read it in public. This antiwar manual will signal to sisters that you're ready to work on the issues that keep us apart.

We *must* end this war. We *can* end this war. I've been a combatant, and now I'm a war correspondent and intelligence analyst, as well as a husband and father. Believe it or not, I'm going to prove to you that it *is* better with the *one* you love.

I know that telling women everything they need to know about their men—what men do and why—and *vice versa* will take us only halfway to peace. The way to a complete and lasting truce that will usher in a new era of black love is open acknowledgment of some difficult truths about ourselves, and willing commitment to making essential changes.

We need to confront tough questions before we can find the answers we seek, such as: "Why don't we trust one another?" and "Where did it all go wrong?" Why are black women and men the walking wounded when it comes to love?

Let's start by listening in to what each side has to say about the other.

How Are Sisters Dealing with Brothers?

When I appeared on a national TV talk show for an episode about black women who refuse to date men of their own race, the onstage panel of women sounded like the Sisters of the KKK! "All a black man can do for me is get my drink on." "All black men want is to hit it and quit it." "Black men are no damn good." And, most bizarre of all, "A white man knows how to treat a woman right." Yeah, they sure treated the sisters right, back on the plantation!

These women represent extreme and exaggerated points of view, but they do reflect a current trend in thinking among black women who want love but are convinced they can't find the love they need from black men. These women have given up on brothers, but these same cynical sisters turn livid whenever they spot a black man with a white woman on his arm. The sight is especially galling if that white woman conforms to the stereotype of the lily-skinned blonde trophy. "As soon as these men get somewhere in life," these sisters grouse, "they do an O. J. and get their white woman!"

Here are more of the sisters' most common complaints about the brothers:

- Black men dog black women as loudly and as frequently as they can.
- This war between us was started by no-account brothers.
- Black men are completely unable to be faithful.
- There are no compatible black men.
- Black men won't and can't communicate.
- Black men are sexually selfish: they want theirs and don't care if you don't get yours.
- They lie.
- They use and abuse you.
- They have children with any female and don't take care of them.

Perhaps the bitterest complaint black women make about black men is that brothers refuse to commit. Commitment is even an issue within long-term relationships that have produced children. On a nearly daily basis, I hear from women who've been in relationships for years, even decades, but the man has dug in his heels and refuses to get married.

When Denise called in to my radio show during a discussion called "Why Buy the Cow When You're Getting the Milk for Free?", she really set it off. Denise had been living with a man for two decades and had borne him four children. Throughout those years, she had begged, pleaded, and cajoled to make it legal. "It is legal," he'd say. "It's common law. Why do we need the white man to give us a piece of paper? I'm here, ain't I? You're my woman."

But she wasn't his *wife*.

You don't have to be Miss Cleo to predict what eventually happened. When he got tired of Denise, her man walked. Not six months passed before he was hitched—in possession of that white man's paper—to a bride half his age!

What's wrong with this picture? Like most sisters stuck with a man who won't commit, Denise would go on and on about how she was fed up and disgusted. But Denise did what most of these angry women do because they feel powerless over the situation—nothing. She forgot that she had choices. Instead, she stayed with her "no-good" man and took the punishment.

"Yeah, your guy was a no-good, manipulating user," I told Denise. "But it takes two to make a bad relationship. You *allowed* him to wipe his feet on you for twenty years, so you have to accept half the responsibility for being treated like a doormat."

With those words, the floodgates opened: the switchboard was deluged with calls from other women who lived with men who refused to walk down the aisle. "These guys are scum," other callers opined. "How can these women be so stupid and passive?" still other callers marveled. "They deserve each other."

"It wasn't me" is another typical male behavior that ranks right under refusal to commit on the lengthy list of sisters' complaints. Brothers activate the overused and tired "It wasn't me" defense whenever they're caught creeping, and no other aspect of the black man's behavior is more infuriating to black women. The line is clever and comical in Shaggy's hit tune inspired by this excuse. In real life, though, "It wasn't me" drives sisters up the wall, and understandably so.

The betrayed woman could be armed with lipstick on his collar: "It wasn't me!" She's clutching a handful of motel room receipts: "It wasn't me!" She's called that mysterious number on his cell phone bill and had a heart-to-heart with the female in question: "It wasn't me!" His underwear is on backward and inside out, even though it was perfectly straight when he stepped out of the house this morning: "It wasn't me!" He's butt naked on the bed with her second cousin, first removed, getting up on his down stroke, and he'll still look her straight in the eye and say, just as cool and calm as you please, "It wasn't me!" I may be exaggerating a bit with that last example, but you get the point. No matter how solid the evidence that Mr. Man has been playing outside his yard, he denies it to the bitter end: "It wasn't me!" His woman never gets her satisfaction, and not only because he refuses to admit he's done wrong.

The main problem is not so much his flagrant infidelity as the fact that most betrayed women rant and rave, but, amazingly, that's all they do. *They choose to hang in there anyway!* Some even boast about their loyalty to men who refuse to be faithful. Ain't that a bitch? These ladies aren't even cashing in on that "fornicate free card" Chris Rock jokes about. At least Rock's somewhat fair-minded; he acknowledges that the least the roving gander owes his faithful goose is a little payback. All jokes aside, though, the problem with this scenario is that too many women stay with their man despite the pain they suffer over his cheating ways. Why? Because they are brainwashed to believe they can't do better.

Lisa, a female client in one of the relationship support groups I run for women, has been with the same man for eighteen years and has borne him two children. Lisa constantly complains about Danny's cheating, even with her so-called girlfriends. One cold February night, she sat in her unheated car outside one woman's apartment building for several hours, staring up at the dark windows of the woman's apartment and waiting for Danny to come out. Finally, Lisa couldn't take the frigid temperature and went home. When Danny sauntered in the door at 6 A.M., she confronted him. Of course, he immediately became angry and insisted, "It wasn't me."

That scene has played out at least fifty to sixty times during the course of their relationship, which, by the way, Danny refuses to make legal. Lisa complains to anyone who'll listen, but she never makes good on her frequent threats to leave him and get on with her life.

"I'm still very proud of myself, because I've stayed completely faithful," Lisa tells me. "But I'm so unhappy, and, worse, our children are beginning to misbehave. I'm sure it's because they know their daddy is running the streets with all kinds of women, so they don't respect me. I pray that God will get me through this."

"God helps those who help themselves," I always respond. "It's time to get yourself out of purgatory."

The last time we talked, I asked one more time, "Why do you stay?"

"What's the point of getting out?" Lisa said in a tired, defeated tone. "My chances of finding a good guy are nil. All black men are the same, so if I went out and got a different one, I'd just land in the same heap of doo-doo. I don't know any black men who are faithful."

Tens, perhaps hundreds of thousands of Lisas are out there. These unhappy, complaining women hang in as willing prisoners of war. An equal number of sisters have grown so cynical about the black man's capacity for love that these women have given up the fight altogether. They are in retreat from the front lines and want nothing to do with the brothers at all.

As if the stereotyping, mistrust, hating, lack of communication, and deadly war games weren't destroying what little mutual trust we have left, the Jesse Jackson scandal became yet another flash point. Here was a religious and moral leader who fathered a child outside his supposedly happy, long-term marriage. Brothers all over the country heaved a collective groan and swore, "Damn! Jesse's gone and done it. We'll be paying for his fun for years to come!" Sisters practically yelped in unison, "We knew it! If this shining example of black leadership—this super brother and number one preacher—can't keep it zipped, what hope is there for the average brother to be faithful! Didn't we tell you? Black men just cannot stay with one woman!"

Sadly, under all that hard, glittering rage is the soft underbelly of the black woman's despair. To put it another way, despite their loud and constant trash talking, sisters are losing the war because they lack confidence. They believe they can't win. They either give up and retreat or settle for whatever they can get, because they have lost faith in themselves and their men.

Now let's move to the opposition's side of the battlefield and check out what black men have to say about black women.

How Are Brothers Dealing with Sisters?

Brothers complain that black women are angry, condescending, suspicious, and manipulating:

- They're never satisfied with the money the black man brings into the home.
- The black woman doesn't understand the day-to-day racism a black man endures.
- Too many sisters are chicken heads who only care about what a brother can buy them.
- Black women are stuck-up, especially if they're educated professionals.
- Sisters, especially the stuck-up ones, say that all they want is a steadfast brother, but they wouldn't know a good brother if he appeared on their doorstep astride a white stallion and bearing roses.
- Sisters really go for the athletes, celebrities, and bad-boy rappers. They want the roughneck who gives them a hard time and treats them cruelly. Then, of course, these women complain all over again that "all black men are dogs."

Successful black women are a favorite target for the black man's animosity, second only to "The Man—who she's probably sleeping with, too!" Professional black women are attacked by black men for being too independent, lacking homemaking skills, being afraid to mess up their hair in bed, refusing to stay up late because of work, refusing to have large broods of children, and not allowing a brother to be "the man" in the relationship.

Together and Miserable

Some of us do manage to dodge the bullets from both sides and get together. Yet even when we couple, most of us continue to battle. Too many of our committed or married couples are locked in vicious cycles of explosive and dysfunctional behavior patterns caused by a near-total breakdown of communication. Many couples living under the same roof and sleeping in the same bed are so angry at each other that they haven't done the nasty in years. Neither partner feels a sense of caring, support, or desire from the other. A wall of pent-up emotion separates them. This estrangement and lack of intimacy and communication is usually created by two conflicting impulses. The man often suffers from a persistent fear of commitment and intimacy, even though he is already committed! His fear goes head to head against the woman's persistent fantasies about being swept off her feet by a black knight in shining armor who pledges undying devotion morning, noon, and night. When couples are locked in this conflict, my role as counselor is to inject a healthy antidote of reality.

Deandra dragged her husband, Richie, into couples counseling because of his sexual disinterest. We all know how much black men enjoy professional counseling! But Deandra insisted. If Richie didn't come with her to see me, she would leave him for good. In our first session, Deandra complained about their lack of intimacy and stated that she suspected her husband no longer loved her. Their lovemaking was extremely infrequent, even though she worked out relentlessly to maintain her shape and tried every trick in Victoria's closet to spark Richie's interest. She even dressed up like Lil' Kim—complete with blond wig, fishnets, and blue contact lenses—but nothing worked. Deandra went on to say that Richie was always cold, angry, and resentful but refused to talk. She simply wanted to know why the fire of their early years had turned to cold ashes.

After she had gone on about their problems for about twenty minutes, I turned to Richie, who'd been slumped in his chair, staring at the floor, throughout Deandra's lengthy tirade.

* * *

"So, Richie, what's up?" I asked.

He shifted uncomfortably in his seat.

"My wife just doesn't understand how stressful the job is," he grumbled.

"Why don't you tell her about it right now?" I invited.

Richie let out a sigh. "I have to deal with the foreman coming down on my case every single day," he began. "He's white, and he just doesn't like us. But I got this union job, and I can't lose it if we want to pay the bills. One time, I did try to talk to my wife about it, but all she could say was, 'Life is unfair; you just have to deal with it and maybe you should check yourself.' " He clenched and unclenched his fist. "It ain't about *me!*"

"How does that make you feel?" I asked.

"I gotta deal with this racist white man on the job busting my balls, and then I come home and my wife tells me to handle it on my own, that it's my fault," he complained. "How would you feel?"

"I guess you're saying you don't feel supported by Deandra," I offered.

"Exactly!" Richie exclaimed. "I love her, but how can she expect me to be there for her when she's not there for me?! How am I supposed to feel like making love to her when she can't even understand what I'm going through day after day? I'm too damn mad with her to make love."

Deandra countered by citing a dozen instances in which she'd had her husband's back. "As far as the job situation goes," she said, "I was just trying to get him to wake up and handle it."

Like so many other black men and women, each partner in this marriage expected the other to "just know" how to fill his or her needs. Deandra wanted sex because it would assure her of Richie's love. For his part, Richie wanted to feel supported, yet he was unable to share his emotional needs. His resentment over his wife's lack of understanding built to a point where he didn't even want to make love.

Like Deandra and Richie, each side in our war has to assume their full 50 percent of the responsibility for our dysfunctional relationships. Each side has to recognize and work through the misunderstandings and misperceptions and the negative behavior patterns that destroy relationships.

Ladies, it isn't about throwing up your hands, doing that little sister neck-wave thing, rolling your eyes, and dismissing the brothers: "I've had it with these triflin' black men. I'm going to get me a nice little white man, even if he has a flat butt!" Or, "I'm going to get with the flava of the month and give my girls a chance."

It's not just about brothers behaving like a pack of dogs. But brothers, it's also not about hitting it and quitting it, refusing to commit because that might involve the work of digging deeper into ourselves and acknowledging our true emotional needs.

It *is* about everyone taking a good, long, hard look in the mirror and asking, "What am I bringing to the equation? How have my issues of self-esteem and my screwed-up upbringing contributed to the less than stellar choices I've made when it comes to relationships?"

Both sides have to withdraw blame so we can figure out what is really going on. And so we must ask: Where is all this anger coming from, and why can't we get our act together?

Post-Traumatic Slavery Disorder

A large part of the answer lies in our past. That's why the next chapter of this book looks at our history to help us understand our present. Post-Traumatic Slavery Disorder—what I refer to as "our" PTSD—has created long-standing complexes about our hair, our complexions, our abilities, our intelligence, and about being together—to name just a few of our many issues. We'll explore why PTSD is the root cause of our war, and we'll take a good, long look at why we're being raised to battle. We'll dissect those little things white folks still say and do that make us "want to holler" and how they contribute to our state of war.

In later chapters, we'll tackle the Complacency-Denial Syndrome that numbs us to our relationship issues and keeps our PTSD alive. We'll describe the ways we can stop blaming each other and start taking responsibility for our actions so we can end the insanity of this war. We'll confront and conquer our stereotypical and self-defeating beliefs and behaviors. Yes. We've bought into those nasty images about who we are and what we're worth, and it's way past time to move beyond all that.

Another chapter delivers on my promise to reveal all the war games—the brothers' secret strategies and the sisters' intelligence-gathering and counterstrategies. I'm not a racist or a prude, and whoever rings your bell is fine with me. But I will discuss why even we don't need to go *there*—that is, turn to partners of other races or our own sex to escape from our problems with the opposite sex of our own race. You will learn how to heal your war-torn relationships and cool down angry partners, and I will prove that brothers—and sisters!—are not naughty by nature, and that we would all be better off if we devoted ourselves to one person.

Finally, we will get into helping our kids form healthy, loving relationships when they are grown. The future of our relationships—and our race—really is in the hands of the generations to come.

You'll discover all this at the same time you'll enjoy real-life love and war stories packed with the same drama, heartbreak, and steamy, roller-coaster love you get in those juicy romance novels stacked on your bedside nightstand.

Let go of the fear that your future holds nothing but a dreary vista of endless lonely nights or empty one-night stands. By the time you finish this book, you will be ready to take all the energy you've tied up in anger, bitterness, fear, and tears and redirect it toward finding the right person for you!

CHAPTER ONE

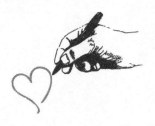

POST-TRAUMATIC SLAVERYDISORDER: THE WAR BEGINS

"I believe most of our brothers are still insecure about themselves because of our past history," a male client named Raymond once observed.

Raymond had come to me after his second marriage failed. Several months into his counseling, he was beginning to recognize how his own thought and behavior patterns had played a role in destroying his relationships, and was wondering where it all began.

"Our insecurity makes it hard for us to face the truth about ourselves," Raymond concluded of black men in general. "A lot of us can't deal with strong women. Black women speak their minds and put up with less crap than other women, whether you like it or not. If you're secure, you should be able to listen to what is being said and evaluate whether or not it applies to you. But we are still too insecure to do that."

Many authorities on African-American history and culture agree with Raymond. These scholars go even further to link many of our destructive relationship patterns to our history as slaves and colonized peoples.

It Started with Slavery

During slavery it was nearly impossible for us to form lasting and healthy relationships. The problem is that, when it comes to getting together for the long term these days, too many of us still act as if the slave master were standing over us with a whip. These carryover mental and behavioral patterns and all the other lingering after-effects of slavery can be described as Post-Traumatic Slavery Disorder, or our PTSD. Every crack of that whip, and the slave master's other cruel acts forced us to react, emotionally and behaviorally, in ways that would protect our sanity, our dignity, and our very lives. Sadly, those emotional and behavioral coping mechanisms have become ingrained over time, even though many of these patterns no longer serve our best interests.

Our PTSD is so prevalent and destructive to our collective mental and physical health that it should be officially recognized as a valid psychological disturbance by the same mainstream institutions that acknowledge post-traumatic stress disorder as a condition requiring treatment. As black people, we also need to acknowledge the reality of our PTSD and do something about it ourselves.

The conventionally recognized condition known as post-traumatic stress disorder is described by the *Diagnostic and Statistical Manual-IV*—the bible for diagnosing all mental health diseases—as an emotional condition, as well as a set of destructive, dysfunctional behaviors that evolves after exposure to a traumatic event over which one has little or no control, such as a car, plane, or train accident, a mugging or rape, or any event that is unexpected and outside the usual human experience.

Symptoms include anxiety, flashback memories of the traumatic event, avoidance of similar situations, nightmares and other sleeping disorders, eating disorders, and paranoia. In many ways, these symptoms help us cope minimally with the trauma, even though these coping mechanisms eventually prove dysfunctional. But these behaviors are all we have to get us through. A person suffering from post-traumatic stress disorder usually needs professional counseling to find more constructive ways of dealing with the trauma.

Post-Traumatic Slavery Disorder fulfills the definition of post-traumatic stress disorder. In fact, Post-Traumatic Slavery Disorder differs from post-traumatic stress disorder only in that our PTSD refers to a single, specific trauma—that of slavery. Also, that one terrible trauma persisted for centuries and was endured by an entire race! Slavery and colonialism created not just post-traumatic stress disorder symptoms, but also shame, degradation, and self-hate.

Imagine the emotional upheaval of being forcibly removed from our land, communities, and families in Africa, and then virtually imprisoned in foreign countries, including America, where we endured brutal and horrific conditions for entire lifetimes. How could we ever recover simply through the passage of time? In fact, we have not recovered. We are suffering from that trauma today, and no aspect of our collective lives as African Americans expresses the devastating effects of our PTSD more dramatically than our male–female relationships.

The damage caused by the extreme and long-lasting injury of slavery is too pervasive and profound even to measure. Our PTSD affects virtually every person of color whose history was blighted by slavery and colonialism. The danger is that if we do not acknowledge and then exorcise the trauma of our PTSD so that it no longer contaminates our hearts, minds, and souls, we are doomed to act out our buried anger and pain through repetitive negative and dysfunctional relationships, especially with each other. Without question, our Post-Traumatic Slavery Disorder is at the root of the current battling between black men and women. Here's why:

We Were Bred Like Animals

From the moment the very first slave was hauled in chains onto the auction block, black men understood that commitment to a woman could bring nothing but heartache and trouble, and black women realized that they could not count on their men. The black man simply did not have the power to protect his woman and children. During slavery, black men and women were not allowed to create lasting partnerships and families. Instead, Africans were bred like prize animals, according to the whims and labor requirements of the slave master. Those slaves who did fall in love and form family units often experienced the pain of seeing them torn apart as children, mothers, and fathers were sold off to distant plantations, with little hope of ever meeting again.

Commitment Meant Trouble

The slave master could force himself sexually on a female slave any time he pleased. And if a black man allowed himself to experience love for a female slave, that love bound both of them to the plantation for life, defeating any motivation for escape.

Remaining emotionally and physically distant and taking on many lovers—that is, ensuring that love and commitment had nothing to do with it—was the black man's only possible psychological and behavioral defense against the certain prospect of emotional pain.

As for the black woman, her best shot at survival was dampening her own emotions and giving in to the whims of the slave master. The only way she could hope for a measure of control over her destiny was through strategic psychology, including turning her rape into a seduction and currying the slave master's favor for her children, herself, and her *real* man.

What man could ever understand and accept that sacrifice? What man would not misinterpret his woman's defense maneuver as collusion with the enemy? And what woman could ever truly accept that her man had allowed her to become a slave in the first place?

Thus were planted the seeds of distrust between black men and women.

We Were Less Than Human

For hundreds of years, we were told by the dominant society that we were not fully human. At one point, we were even counted in the official census as three-fourths of a human! In fact, the only way we could gain self-esteem was through fulfilling the slave master's demands—by being good workers and good breeders who produced as many new slaves as possible. If you are told something about yourself many times over a lengthy period of time, you inevitably take in that message about who you are and what you're worth. That's how we were brainwashed. We internalized the slave master's degrading view of us as less than human and came to view ourselves as inferior. Once we'd absorbed that destructive view of ourselves as individuals and as a race, our behavior came to reflect that perception.

Many of us also bought into the master as our father figure, and the notion that we, as obedient children, had to please him. This is a common psychological phenomenon known as the Stockholm syndrome, in which a kidnapped or oppressed person learns to depend on her or his captor for survival.

Buried Wounds

Our slavery-induced low self-esteem keeps us in emotional shackles because we are still repeating the same negative behaviors we evolved in order to cope with that self-image problem. Why? Because we haven't fully accepted where our negative self-image and behavior patterns come from and what we are doing to keep that negativity going. As a people, we have never made a concerted effort to understand and heal slavery's destructive effects on our relationships. No wonder we can't get along!

Only when we can free ourselves of our PTSD and our negative self-images and stereotypes—as well as the anger, pain, and fear these self-concepts create—will we finally be able to come together in love.

You may object that slavery days have been done and gone for nearly a century and a half. Whenever I give talks and workshops on relationships, I can count on someone to say, "Isn't it time for black men and women to get over it and clean up their acts? How can what happened so long ago during slavery still affect how we relate to each other today? PTSD is just some psychobabble excuse for tired behavior with each other!"

True, slavery is over in America, but we have yet to get over it. The experience lives on in our bodies, hearts, minds, and souls, and the racism we experience every day helps keep the trauma alive and tear our families apart.

Let me break it down even further. Here are five proofs that our PTSD is the biggest threat to our relationships today:

Unresolved emotional pain doesn't just go away

Someone suffers from post-traumatic stress disorder because he or she has internalized a traumatic experience. This means that the experience ended, but the emotional pain caused by the trauma is not over. It hasn't been worked through and resolved, so the trauma remains trapped inside, where it colors that person's every emotion, belief, and behavior. The only way to become free of the trauma and cure post-traumatic stress disorder is, one, by acknowledging the trauma and the pain it causes; and, two, gaining a healthy understanding, either through therapy, counseling, or dialogue with an empathetic and insightful person. Now, how many black people do you know who have undergone therapy in order to heal their Post-Traumatic Slavery Disorder? In fact, how many black people do you know who even recognize that concept, let alone discuss it in conversation?

Our emotional wounds are still repressed deep inside and, for the most part, unacknowledged by our conscious minds. This is why our wounds haven't healed and our relationships suffer. You can never completely deny any powerful experience or deep emotion, no matter how much you act as though you just don't care by pushing that emotion out of your conscious awareness. Unacknowledged emotions always struggle to be acknowledged, and they never give up. This is why the PTSD we suppress keeps rearing its ugly head and fighting for recognition. It "speaks" to us through our pain and the dysfunctional ways in which we behave toward each other.

We learn from our parents

We learn how to interact with the opposite sex as children by observing how our parents relate to each other or to other partners. Of course, our parents learned from their parents, who learned from theirs, and so it goes—which takes us right back to slavery days, when close, committed relationships were a threat rather than a safe haven. As I've already noted, Big Massa may be retired to the ole plantation in the sky, but the behaviors we created to defend us from his cruelties are alive and well. They live in Great Grandma's observation that "all men are dawgs" and Great Grandpa's dismissal of "sneaky bitches." Those wholesale disses of each other reflect not only what Great Grandma and Great Grandpa learned at their mamas' and papas' knees, but also our entire history in America. Children don't know any better. They simply absorb the viewpoints of their elders. As they grow, they act from those viewpoints and observed adult behaviors, then pass all of that on to their own youth. Through the generations, we've been raising our children to battle each other, because we've never stopped defending ourselves against Big Massa.

We've been genetically programmed to battle!

My experience as a psychologist leads me to believe that many of the dysfunctional ways of relating we developed during slavery actually became genetic. Through enough repetition, behaviors can become hard-wired into our brains, forming actual neural pathways—in much the same way that a computer is programmed to spit out the same information over and over. These "programmed" responses are then passed on to future generations. Over the centuries, the unhealthy behaviors created by the conditions of slavery have given us an actual genetic disposition toward dysfunctional relationships.

Slavery may be over, but racism lives on

Some racist words and deeds are as bold as day. More often, though, it's the little things that count. No matter how thick your skin, it's nearly impossible to ignore the subtle insults we receive on a daily basis from the white majority. That everyday brand of racism simply reinforces the emotional distress and destructive behaviors associated with Post-Traumatic Slavery Disorder. Our present is conspiring with our past to keep us stuck in an unhealthy emotional state in which we release our pain on the most convenient targets— each other.

Romance without finance has no chance!

Educational and economic inequities are all-too-real fallout from Post-Traumatic Slavery Disorder and the pressures of past and present-day racism. Economic issues are the number one reason why couples of any race can't get it together. If there's no money, love fights extra hard to survive. Day-to-day grinding poverty wears away at the strongest love. With black people still poised on the lowest rung of America's economic ladder, our view of each other as fail-ures—and therefore as less attractive relationship prospects than partners of other races!—is reinforced.

The deteriorating quality of black men and women's relationships clearly results from the ways in which we learned to cope with slav-ery. Yet our PTSD doesn't take us off the hook. Ultimately, we bear the responsibility for reinforcing our PTSD by staying stuck in dys-functional ways of thinking and behaving.

Let's take a closer look at the more common PTSD-associated syndromes and behaviors we need to lose, because they are destroy-ing our chances for more loving relationships.

Acting Out Sexually

Slavery was not only an emotional and physical crime against black people and humanity overall; it was also a brutal sex crime. It was rape—physically, psychologically, and spiritually. Our men and women were sexually exploited in every way possible, from the lit-eral rape of our women to enforced breeding with partners of the master's choice. Our sexual/physical abuse has affected us in ways similar to other victims of sexual abuse who take in the message of the rape and come to use their sexuality to define themselves. Those of us who have bought into society's view that all black people have to offer is sexual and physical power, base their behavior on a warped sense of sexuality. That dysfunctional sexuality has become the way some of us define our self-worth and our relationships. We use sex as a weapon. We use sex to help us feel better about ourselves. We even use sex to keep us from becoming truly intimate.

I often hear black men reduce black women to what's between their legs, while black women reduce black men to what they can do for them in bed.

If you can't commit on a healthy emotional level, what else is left but to act out what you know best—sex? For some, sex is the only way they relate to a partner, but if knocking boots is the sole basis of a relationship, sex is just a release valve. Sex is no longer a way to create and strengthen an intimate connection. If a man has more than one "release valve," you can be sure he's also using these sexual conquests to boost his ego. After all, what did the black man have back in slavery days? He didn't have the right to protect his woman and children, to earn a living, own property, even to read or write. And if he did sex well, why not turn that negative into a positive? Why not take pride in his prowess? The same could be said of the female slave. If she was used and abused by the master, why not cultivate the skill of sexual manipulation in order to conquer the slave master and protect herself and her family? Back then, sexual prowess and manipulation were means of survival, but many of us still believe that they are our only talents. That warped point of view lies at the core of a destructive repertoire of limited sex-based relationship behaviors that are unhealthy for us as individuals and as a race. Let's take a look at how this plays out:

Buck and the Breeder

We all know a Buck when we meet one, and by now we understand where Buck's penis-waving comes from: our PTSD. "The white man may hold the political and money power, but I got the penis power," Buck is saying. I'm not about to tell you that sexual prowess is bad. Black men probably deserve their reputation as studly lovers. The problem comes in when you believe that's the *only* power you have. Sexual skill is wonderful, but basing relationships on between-the-sheets talent is limiting. Physical intimacy alone cannot build a healthy, close relationship that will nurture you and your partner in an emotionally gratifying way.

Of course, all the Bucks out there reason that they have to share their gifts with many women because there aren't enough strong black men to go around. These brothers claim that it would be selfish if they didn't share "this much man" with more than one woman.

Raoul was a typical example of a Buck who was forcing his wife, Cynthia, to be a breeder. Raoul was never home. Cynthia had even found a few mysterious phone calls on his cell phone bill, and other telltale signs of her husband's cheating. Of course, Raoul stoutly denied infidelity and countered Cynthia's accusations with intimidating temper tantrums. Cynthia finally took a stand and threatened to leave if he didn't come with her to counseling.

After a few therapy sessions, we still weren't getting anywhere, so I suggested that each of them also meet with me individually.

Raoul was much more forthcoming when we were alone. In fact, he figured that as a brother I'd understand where he was coming from.

"Listen man, I've been with my wife for eight years, and you know a man's got to do what a man's got to do," he told me. "I can't be with the same woman all that time. Not with all these honeys out there just begging for it. I have to spread it around. What has Cynthia got to complain about? I pay the bills. I take care of her and the kids, and I give her the good wood a couple of times a week. What's her problem? Lots of sisters would love to be in her shoes. Why can't I have fun on my private time? I need you to tell me how to handle Cynthia."

Unfortunately, this Buck spoke for too many black men. Cynthia was not his lover or his partner. She was the means to his ends: having children and a well-run household. Cynthia's feelings and the quality of their relationship were not factors to be considered. Distracted by the ego boosts he got from his many affairs, Raoul was completely unaware that his behavior was slowly but surely eroding his emotional connection with his wife. Cynthia was just another female to be squeezed into his busy schedule.

Once we'd addressed some of the issues in their dysfunctional marriage, Cynthia refused to accept her limited role in their relationship. Yet many black women willingly take on the role of servant/breeder/mammy. Like Buck, these women view themselves in a one-dimensional mirror. Of course, the Breeder is also a legacy of slavery, when female slaves were a means of increasing the master's property. The Buck is brainwashed by PTSD to think that all he's got going for himself is his penis, while the Breeder believes that all she has to offer is a womb in which to make a baby that will tie a man to her for life. Unfortunately, after many Bucks make deposits in a sperm bank, they feel their job is done and withdraw further support. In fact, they usually brag about how wide and far they've scattered their seed, without ever taking into account their complete failure to be real men and raise and support those children.

I'm also dismayed by the increasing numbers of young black girls I see at my clinic whose PTSD expresses itself in their assumption that having a child at age fifteen or sixteen is a common rite of passage. Who are these girls' role models? Often the role models are their own mothers and grandmothers. Even when these adult women warn their daughters and granddaughters over and over about the difficulties of single parenthood at an early age, the older women's example suggests to their girls that they'll be able to manage, too.

Many young women have no clue why they're having babies in the first place. They offer vague reasons, the most common being, "I want someone to love and love me"—clear evidence that self-esteem issues are the core reason for babies to have babies. If these young mothers believed in themselves and their futures, they would not tie themselves down so early in life with the responsibilities of a child. Their inability to believe in themselves as potential movers and shakers who could make a mark in the world, or even as wives in loving and equal partnerships, also colors how men view them. Prospective mates take one look at the baby on the hip and the toddler tugging at the skirt, and dismiss these young women as Breeders.

Punany Power

Other women, especially younger women, believe the best they can do—given black men's shoddy behavior and the unfavorable black-man-to-black-woman population ratio—is to flip the script and work their own equivalent of penis power. I call it punany power, to borrow a Caribbean term for female genitalia. In fact, many of these women will do just about anything to prove their P-power is better than the competition's. It's all about the Benjamins anyway, because these girls have given up on true love and turned into sexual mercenaries. Of course, punany power is also linked to slavery days, when black females were viewed as sex objects for the master's pleasure. The prettiest slaves may have attracted more unwanted play, but in some instances they also won privileges. They may have been sexual victims and hostages, but they could also use sex to gain some semblance of control over the master and even their own destinies. Throughout time, all women—regardless of race and ethnicity—have been raped and exploited by men, but women of color have suffered the hardest lessons of sexual survival. Black men learned to use their strength and their penises, while black women learned to use their feminine wiles and sexuality.

Punany power is on display today in the R&B, hip-hop, and reggae videos all over TV. It's "for sale" at the local club. Again, the emphasis on sex as the sole connection between men and women is a lingering aftereffect of an outmoded survival strategy, but it cannot lead to strong, close bonds between our men and women. And when "hotties" age, what happens to self-esteem without the slamming body to maintain morale? Throughout their youth, these women attracted men who wanted them for their physical attributes only, which means they've endured one failed relationship after another. Those types of men always move on to hunt down other conquests. Very attractive women who rely on punany power often find themselves older and alone and wondering why.

Masking Feelings

When you relate to others on the basis of sex, you naturally suppress softer, more vulnerable emotions. While both genders are capable of protecting their more tender emotions, masking feelings tends to be more a male problem. Men in general are socialized to suppress their sensitivity so everyone will perceive them as manly.

"Rambro"

Black men, in particular, fear being regarded as "soft," that is, emotionally weak and like a female. During slavery, many black men swallowed their pain and humiliation by acting stony and "tough." We see that lingering PTSD coping tactic in brothers who present to the world an unfeeling, macho mask that hides and protects their fear and hurt, even their tender love. The only powerful emotions many black men are willing to show the world are so-called strong ones: anger and rage. These men are really hurting and understandably so, but they fear that if they were to risk revealing their vulnerability, at best they would be laughed at and scorned. At worst, they'd be destroyed.

Of course, men who cannot expose their vulnerability are so emotionally bottled up, they have difficulty saying, "I love you" or even being physically tender, not only with their partners, but also with their children.

Part of the problem is that black men are still objects of contempt. They remain an endangered species in this society and are the least empowered men of any race. In fact, black men believe their status in America at large doesn't even measure up to the black woman's. In fact, studies prove this perception isn't true. What *is* true, though, is that black men *believe* black women are allowed to exercise more power in mainstream society.

"Sambo"

Again, masking feelings was a necessary, often effective survival strategy back on the plantation. "Rambros" adopted a stoic, macho facade, but many other black men hid their true feelings under an at-

39

titude of complete submission. These men presented to the world a mild, subservient, and nonthreatening face—the "Sambo." Underneath the mask of compliance, these Sambos seethed with rage over having to play their pathetic, shuffling role. Playing Sambo is now recognized as a coping mechanism that sometimes included sly, coded gestures that signaled to other slaves how slick Sambo was really "getting over." Yet even when Sambo got over, he paid a stiff price for his defense. Sambo paved over the same pain suffered by Rambro.

Sambos were equally poor candidates for nurturing relationships. They may have acted like the most jovial, yes-sir/no-sir fellas for the outside world, but once they shut their front door and were safe at home, these nice guys often turned into raging bullies who released the pain and pressure-cooker rage by lashing out at their close ones. Few full-out Sambos exist today, but many black men still shift between two personalities: one tailored for the white world, the other for "us." These men also suffer because they lose contact with their true selves. Unable to inhabit their natural identity all the time, they cannot establish a genuine relationship with someone else.

Sisters Doing It for Themselves . . . and Everyone Else

During slavery, the black woman often had to take care of everything on her own because her man was not allowed to assert husbandly or fatherly responsibilities. Many black women today still believe they have to take care of everything, and these overburdened women often dismiss all black men as useless, incompetent fools. "I can do better on my own," they tell themselves—and each other, especially during those group grouses about "useless brothers."

It's hard to blame overcompensating sisters for their bitterness, especially when they have "bred" for more than one man who's let them down, were raised in a fatherless home, or witnessed their mothers or close relatives and friends repeatedly abused or abandoned by lovers or the fathers of their children. In fact, some overcompensating women insist they want nothing at all to do with a black man or even a family.

Other black women do marry and stay with a black man, but they never dream of demanding a fifty-fifty partnership. They stay with their men but they give up on a genuine relationship. These sisters simply decide from the get-go that they have to take care of everything, and they often wind up emasculating their husbands in the process.

Not surprisingly, many of these sisters walk around with a giant chip on their shoulders. Who wouldn't be angry if they'd convinced themselves that they have to take care of everything because no one will help? Again, these women are often justified to some extent, but they're also throwing out the baby with the bath water. Not all black men are worthless, shiftless, and irresponsible; and many of these women don't even realize that they can expect, ask for, and receive help from a man and enjoy fifty-fifty love.

Giving up on black men, whether refusing to deal with them altogether or not expecting them to live up to their obligations, only leads to personal pain and our disaster as a race.

The Complexion Complex

For many of us, the standards of attractiveness set by the slave master still rule. Within the plantocracy, light-skinned slaves enjoyed more status because of their obvious associations with the slave master. A light complexion and "good" hair meant that you were the son or daughter of the master or, at the very least, of an overseer. It sometimes even provided entry to the Big House, where work was slightly less grueling than in the fields, and certainly of a higher rank. That complexion complex may be one of the most stubborn carryovers from slavery days, and our PTSD has caused us to spin off many variations on its theme of self-rejection.

Darker-skinned slaves very quickly learned that they were inferior to their mixed-race peers. Dark-skinned men and women were viewed as "primitive," driven by animal sexuality. This point of view was so aggressively forced on us that we finally internalized the slaver's contempt for African beauty. We began to view "good hair," "fine features," and light skin as superior and beautiful. The same prejudices attached themselves to the width of our noses, the size of our behinds, and the fullness of our lips. African features became a source of shame and ugliness. This introduced a divisive element into the slave population, where dark- and light-skinned slaves viewed each other with suspicion. Dark-skinned slaves were envious of the light-skinned slaves' position and favor, and light-skinned slaves bought into the master's contempt for the purely African. Even siblings within the same slave family were affected if some children were fathered by a slave while others were fathered by the master.

Those distorted perceptions endure today. The many stereotypes that arise from our issues around complexion shade and other features are land mines in our war between the sexes. Light-skinned folk may look down on dark-complexioned people, but that script is flipped by darker-complexioned people who sneer at light-skinned black people, calling them "white," "stuck up," and "not really black." As a result, we not only suffer from the stereotypes and racism inflicted on us by others, but we also mirror those distorted views in the ways in which we treat each other.

As ludicrous as those prejudices are, they linger on in our minds as part of our PTSD that is destroying our relationships.

Dating Exclusively Outside Our Race

"It has always amazed me that black men are the only race to talk about how they hate their own women and don't want to date us," Amanda complained during a women's group session. "Have they forgotten that they all came from a black woman's womb? Do you ever hear white men spitting out such venom toward white women? Who taught us how to love and get along with each other? Our parents. Who did our parents learn from? Their parents. And we can track it back to being transported to this country and sold as slaves for the white man's pleasure."

Of course, we all know love has no color, but when black people—men or women—refuse to date anyone of their own race, that is a flagrant sign of PTSD-induced self-esteem issues. Such a person is also giving up on our future as a race in this country. Black men and women who claim that partners of the other race "treat me better" are usually escapists who don't want to take a long, hard look at their own motives. Refusing to consider a brother or sister reflects a self-hate that's expanded into hate of your own kind. Of course, it all goes back to the slave master's contempt that we absorbed and made our own.

Those of us who eject our own race from our personal dating pools may also believe on some level that partners of a different race are potential "saviors." "White women will give us more class." "Asian women will obey us." "White men will treat us better and give us access to a better life." For some men, dating white women is a way to get back at the master or gain greater status.

Victimizing the Victim

Americans were shocked by recent news accounts of Bosnian wives, sisters, and daughters who were killed by male relatives because these women had been raped by Serb fighters. These murderous husbands, brothers, and fathers couldn't handle the dishonor to their families. This is an extreme instance of a common human phenomenon: "blaming the victim" for his or her own suffering. Many black men are unaware that they blame black women, on some level, for being raped by the master. Of course, the blame comes down even harder on those women who willingly entered into liaisons with white men in order to survive. Black men may be aware that their women had little choice, but deep down inside, a little voice keeps whispering, "It was her fault." Many brothers are still simmering with rage over the rape of their black women by the white slave masters, and, whether they know it or not, these brothers have fallen into the trap of victimizing the victim. The widespread attitude of distrust many brothers hold toward today's sisters is, at least in part, a carryover from the male slave's suspicion that his woman colluded in her own rape, even if she may have done so in order to protect herself, her man, and their children. It's not surprising that most contemporary black men's blood pressure soars whenever they spot a sister accompanied by a white man: visions of that primal rape scene dance in their heads. And when the anger rises up, it has to go somewhere. More often than not, the anger spills out onto that black woman and her white man, then onto all other black women as well. After all, they, too, could be getting it on with the white man!

On the other hand, some black women unconsciously blame their men for not preventing slavery. Ironically, these women can so resent the black man's powerlessness, that white men become the saviors who can change black women's destinies.

We have to keep in mind that many of these dysfunctional beliefs are unconscious and that the behaviors created by these belief systems were originally coping mechanisms that ensured our survival during slavery. But coping came at a tremendous cost in terms of our psychological well-being, and we're still paying. In later chapters, we will deal with the effects of our PTSD on our relationships, and how we can heal. We'll explore where we typically go wrong and why. You will understand why those of us who believe we are players are actually fumblers. You will learn all the ways we keep the war going and how to stop the madness by developing healthier ways of thinking and behaving.

But before we can begin to resolve all the issues caused by our PTSD and create deeper, more supportive love connections, we first need to explore the role of our complacency and denial in keeping our PTSD behaviors alive and sabotaging our relationships.

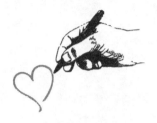

CHAPTER TWO

THE COMPLACENCY-DENIAL SYNDROME: KEEPING OUR PTSD ALIVE

Our PTSD has created desperate, lonely, angry black women and callous, commitment-phobic black men. The damage doesn't stop there. Our PTSD continues to have an impact on almost every aspect of our lives. It is a well-known truth that unhealthy relationships and relationship patterns can lead to all sorts of emotional and physical problems. The reverse is also true. Improved health is one of many benefits marriage confers upon men. According to research done by Steven L. Nock, a University of Virginia sociology professor, married men have better jobs, earn more money, give more to charity, and attend church more frequently than their single counterparts. Nock and others conclude that steady companionship yields significant benefits, physically and psychologically, especially to men. Yet destructive relationships can be lethal to women. The first intimations that a woman's health might be affected by her marital relationship came a decade or so ago, when researchers from the Framingham Heart Study concluded that although married men live longer than their single counterparts, single women tend to outlive women who chose to wed.

When researchers took a closer look at the issue and considered the effects of good and bad marriages on health, they found that women were much more vulnerable than men to the bumps in the road.

For example, according to a study published in the *Journal of the American Medical Association,* women who had suffered a heart attack were three times more likely to sustain a second attack if they were in a stressful relationship than single women or women in an unstressful relationship. Researchers found that work stress, on the other hand, had no impact on the heart health of the women in the study.

All this makes the need to face down our PTSD and eliminate its harmful effects even more urgent. Our survival depends on it. Working out our PTSD won't be easy, but perseverance, honesty, and determination will see us through. The first steps in any process are often the most difficult. In this case, the first step toward confronting and resolving our PTSD is accepting the reality that we do suffer from serious relationship difficulties. That also involves acknowledging that our PTSD exists. It also means that we must acknowledge our pain. If we are ever going to get it together and find the love we need, we must face the fact that we are hurting and that our hurt runs deep! Defeating our PTSD also means we must admit that our PTSD is the reason we are the least likely group to get it together and love each other. Our PTSD is the reason why divorce, single-parent homes, and loneliness are more likely to afflict us than any other race. Here's the six-million-dollar answer to a question we're afraid to ask: "Why can't we get along?" Our PTSD is the answer, as well as the reason why we won't even ask.

Whoever said ignorance is bliss was dead wrong. Confusion and ignorance are painful. We may feel as if we're getting by on the day-to-day, but the victims of our confusion and ignorance are strewn all over the killing fields of our war, and every minute of every day, relationship time bombs are blowing up.

We should declare a national emergency, call for government-funded studies to help us discover what's going on within our marriages and families. Our relationship woes are hurting us not just as singles and couples, but also as mothers, fathers, and as a race. Our economic and civil rights gains have been significant, but if we are miserable, caught outside the comfort zone offered by healthy relationships, all the money and social status in the world mean little or nothing. If we cannot break the cycle of pain created by our PTSD, our children will be doomed to suffer as much, if not more. If we allow this to happen, we will have destroyed not only our relationships but also all the economic and social gains our ancestors sacrificed so much to win.

If we do not recognize the trouble we're in, we cannot summon up enough motivation and drive to make the necessary changes to improve our romantic and social interactions.

There is good news: the quality of our relationships *is* under our control. We can create a more stable existence, happier love lives, and exemplary marriages. All it takes is commitment to work on healing our PTSD—to healing the wounds that affect each of us as individuals, and the wounds that affect us all.

Where do we begin? For each of us, the work starts at home, by understanding and addressing our own personal issues. Believe me, as you read further, you will be amazed at the destructive path our Post-Traumatic Slavery Disorder has cut in your life. You will come to understand that our PTSD has blinded you to your relationship issues and the emotional pain they are causing. It's almost as if our PTSD has a will to survive and we help keep it going through our complacency and denial.

Human beings in general prefer the comfort of the familiar, however painful that rut may be. It's the same with our PTSD. Despite the dysfunction and pain it causes, we have grown comfortable in the familiarity of our dysfunctional ways of viewing each other and relating to each other, and we've numbed ourselves to the pain of our failure to connect. Ignorance may not be bliss, but in this case, it's a worn-out, sprung armchair we've settled into, and we're too lazy to get out.

Wave Your Hands in the Air; Shake 'Em Like You Just Don't Care: The Complacency-Denial Syndrome

After many years practicing therapy with hundreds if not thousands of black couples, I've concluded that many of us suffer from a state of mental paralysis I call Complacency-Denial Syndrome, or CDS. This syndrome is not listed in the *DSM-IV—Revised,* the reference book of psychiatric diagnoses, but CDS is all too real, and this syndrome runs rampant among our people.

CDS includes two phases. Phase one is complacency. Complacency means that, no matter how bad our relationship problems, we accept the situation as part of life and how we have to live. Complacency means we've given up, and we view our dismal lot as normal. Numb to our emotional pain and unhappiness, we don't question what we can do about it. It's as if the pain that was once sharp and distressing has settled down into a chronic ache we can live with. Our spouse's cheating and drinking, which used to cause such distress and jeopardize the relationship, has become a familiar problem that's moved from crisis mode to a "cross I have to bear."

This is Phase One CDS—complacency, when change is possible if one or both partners reach a breaking point where they feel they just cannot live any longer with the chronic problem.

Terrie and Leron had been married over fifteen years. During all that time, not one year passed in which Leron was not involved in an extramarital relationship. After the first couple of years of fighting and her empty threats to leave, Terrie resigned herself to the fact that her husband would never be faithful. She convinced herself that she was lucky to have a husband at all. Her girlfriends had grown so desperate for "good black men" that they'd been forced to travel all the way back to Africa to find husbands and bring them home to start a new life. As long as Leron was home before midnight on weekdays and by 2 A.M. on weekends, Terrie could grin and bear it. Was she happy? No. But was she married? Yes. That was most important.

Terrie's complacency came to a crashing end when her husband gave her a case of genital herpes he'd caught from a new girlfriend. The herpes virus also caused a frightening and painful bout of shingles that landed Terrie in the hospital for over two weeks. Terrie finally sought therapy. Her illness had forced her to realize that complacent acceptance of Leron's behavior was neither emotionally nor physically healthy. After months of treatment, Terrie developed the resolve to stand up for her rights as a wife and person. She demanded that her husband be faithful to the marriage. That snapped Leron to attention, and he stopped his affairs for a few months, but he soon picked up with another home girl. Finally, Terrie knew she had to kick him to the curb.

Most of us are like Terrie—stuck in Phase One. We can still wake from our slumber and do something about our relationship misery.

Phase Two, the denial aspect of CDS, presents a tougher challenge. Denial is much more dangerous, because it offers less opportunity to break out of the dysfunctional relationship malaise. If not challenged, chronic complacency—which usually includes some elements of denial, since these two phases are not completely distinct—can turn into full-fledged denial.

Complacency allows us to tolerate relationship pain. Denial sets in once we've convinced ourselves that the *circumstances* causing our pain don't even exist. Once we can't even recognize the dysfunction of our relationship pattern, we persuade ourselves that we're not even in emotional pain. When we're complacent, we acknowledge that our situation is negative, but we don't believe we can change it. When we move past complacency and into denial, we become oblivious both to the problems with our situation and to our pain. For example, a person who's moved into the denial phase of CDS may refuse to believe that his or her partner has a drinking problem, even though everyone else recognizes that the person is a stone-cold drunk. The alcoholic's partner also denies that he or she is suffering, but that pain is also evident to everyone else. Yet the pain always struggles to be recognized. That pain may not even express itself as emotional discomfort—as depression, anxiety, or anger. Physical symptoms such as headaches, digestive disturbances, lethargy, hives, and other bodily conditions can be evidence of a person's denied suffering. People who deny their emotional pain often sense something is wrong. They feel vaguely unhappy and suspect that in some way they are not fully inhabiting their lives, but they don't know exactly what's wrong. They fail to recognize the real source of their discomfort.

Harriet had been running to doctors for years because of her gastrointestinal problems: chronic indigestion, a burning throat, and an inability to digest her food, especially if she ate any time after six in the evening. During her last middle-of-the-night visit to the emergency room, a doctor began questioning Harriet about her marriage. At first, she was insulted and couldn't understand what the connection was between her physical symptoms and his intrusive questions about her private life. Her doctor gently explained that many women he'd seen with similar symptoms also had severe relationship issues that they'd failed to identify as important problems. Since these women denied their emotional issues, it was difficult, if not impossible, for them to connect their medical conditions with their re-lationship problems. The doctor gave Harriet the wake-up call she needed.

Harriet accepted that she was not happy in her relationship with her boyfriend, who was emotionally distant and physically unloving. As a matter of fact, they had not been intimate for the past three years of their five-year relationship. Somehow she had reached a stage of denial in which she'd convinced herself that she wasn't feeling lonely and physically abandoned. She had even told herself that sex was not important for some relationships, including her own. Talking about the details of her relationship with her boyfriend in a therapeutic setting helped Harriet realize that she had moved from complacency to denial. She allowed herself to experience her sadness, isolation, and rage for the first time. She understood that her denial involved "swallowing" these feelings, and that those feelings were struggling for recognition by literally burning their way up her stomach and throat. After several therapy sessions and sharing her feelings with her boyfriend, Harriet got far more relief than from any antacid.

Emotions always strive to be recognized, and they're always dropping clues through various aspects of your life in an ongoing attempt to attract your attention. They are driven to gain acknowledgment, acceptance, and peace. Read through this checklist of symptoms to help you figure out whether or not you have sunk into complacency or even denial about problems with your relationship or relationship patterns:

- Chronic irritability. We often displace anger over our situation onto less important and threatening road bumps in our lives. Instead of expressing anger at our partner, we insult the bus driver or a casual acquaintance.

- Depression. Depression can express itself as pervasive sadness, without your knowing why you're sad. Depressed people often feel tired, hopeless, uninterested, and unmotivated.
- Forgetfulness. So much energy can be expended protecting complacency-denial that not enough is left to focus on the day-to-day details of your life.
- Isolation. Again, the struggle to maintain complacency-denial leaves little energy to engage with other people.

CDS Is Infectious

We've looked at how CDS supports our PTSD by keeping us stuck, unable to take the first steps toward recognizing our dysfunctional relationship patterns and rehabilitating ourselves. The damage doesn't stop there. CDS is so insidious that it's actually infectious. Once we've passed through CDS Phase One (complacency) and onto CDS Phase Two (denial), we begin living in a daze and accepting the terms of our dysfunctional relationship.

If we have a partner, he can be affected as well, because we're allowing him to take a free pass from confronting his share of responsibility for the relationship woes. This is called enabling, or facilitating, someone else's negative behaviors. That partner views your complacency and denial as permission to keep on with the negative behavior. The cheating spouse or the emotionally abusive boyfriend reasons that since he has not been confronted about inappropriate behavior, it's just fine to continue misbehaving. In many cases, the license to act out even becomes permission to step up the bad behavior a notch or two. The unfaithful partner may stop cheating on the sly and begin doing it openly, bringing affairs right into the marriage bed instead of sneaking around at the local motel. Even worse, the emotionally abusive boyfriend may believe he can get physical.

Jonathan was extremely controlling of his wife, Anna. It started with not allowing her to go out with her girlfriends unless he was present. Anna didn't even put up a fight, at least not hard enough for Jonathan to notice. Soon, he was ordering her to report home immediately after work by 5:30 P.M. Anna could not hang out with coworkers for even a few moments or go shopping. If she arrived home later than 5:30, she had to give an explanation and present a copy of her time card for the following week. Jonathan should never have got away with these behaviors, but Anna was tied up in a serious knot of CDS—complacency and denial. Her low self-esteem caused her to accept the unacceptable, so she offered no resistance to her husband's increasingly controlling behavior. Unchecked emotional abuse soon developed into physical abuse as Jonathan began slapping Anna around every time she failed to follow his mandates exactly to the letter of his law. One night, a neighbor overheard her cries and called the police. Jonathan spent a few days in jail and was placed on probation with the condition of therapy. Anna was placed in a safe house for victims of domestic violence. She also received therapy to help her deal with her self-esteem issues as well as her complacency and denial about her relationship. Through interacting with her support group, Anna finally realized what she'd allowed to happen, and she left Jonathan for good.

As you can see, the Complacency-Denial Syndrome is bad business not just for our relationships but also for our physical welfare. It also spells disaster for our well-being as a race. Before we tackle ways in which we can wake up from CDS, let's gain a better understanding of its historical context and origins. We can't begin to solve the problem if we don't know how it began.

The History of CDS

CDS originated with slavery because we were forced to accept—even deny—our situation in order to endure it. After all, what choice did we have? We either complied or died. But CDS didn't end with slavery; it even escalated during the postslavery years along with our growing involvement in the church. Our black churches, the pillars of our community, were towers of strength that helped us get through the chaos of the postslavery era—its legacy of hate and our relegation to the lowly slot of third-class citizenship. Our churches taught us to fight racism and prejudice with the mighty power of our love. Our churches taught us that if we could not get justice here on earth, our suffering would be rewarded in heaven. This message forged a coping mechanism that has served us admirably, religious and heathen alike, for many decades. The problem is that we took the message and ran with it. We became a race of martyrs who take pride in our martyrdom. We were used, abused, flogged, and hung out to dry, and we *still* survived as a race and culture, so that abuse became ennobling. We became the "wretched of the earth," as the famed black psychiatrist Dr. Fritz Fanon described us in his landmark book of the same title.

Pride is wonderful, but "holding our head high" despite the constant pain and humiliation of racism has gone overboard and become complacency and denial about our dysfunctional relationships. If the color of our skin means we have suffered injustice, some of us then reason that part of that necessary suffering entails tolerating the unfairness of relationship dysfunction. The pain of bad relationships and racism has become so entrenched and familiar that it's become expected—it's our lot, an inevitable part of being black. Like Billie Holiday, we greet that pain as a familiar companion: "Good morning, heartache, old friend; sit right on down."

For some of us, pain is our redemption. I've written a brief composition that reflects the pain-as-redemption attitude in what I hope is a humorous way. I call it "The Black Folks' Relationship Prayer":

"O Lawd, I know my time on this earth is about suffering and bad relationships. I know, O Lawd, that you've handed me this burden of pain and misfortune to make me a better person and more deserving of wonderful relationships with the angels in Heaven. Thank you for the pain, O Lawd."

That satirical prayer illustrates the true insanity of complacency and denial. The pain and torment of dysfunctional relationships are not normal, and they are not purifying. The stoic ability to withstand pain that serves us so well in coping with racism has given us an overly high tolerance for bad relationships. That's plain wrong and unhealthy.

Over and over again, Rose found herself involved with men who were otherwise involved. She didn't believe this pattern had anything to do with a possible emotional issue, and she even came to view her situation as an exalted destiny. "Sometimes the vibe is just there with a man," she told me. "It's not like I plan it, but when the stars are right, you just have to go for it, even if he is committed. You never know what will happen." Yet the same thing happened every time she connected with a "destined" lover. He'd play a while with Rose, then bounce right back to his wife or girlfriend.

The first time Rose made a connection with a committed man was at her health club in Pittsburgh, Pennsylvania. As she was running on the treadmill, Rose felt someone's eyes on her. She glanced quickly to her left and caught a blur of glistening, cinnamon brown muscles. Simon flashed Rose a charming smile. A surge of heat and excitement gripped Rose's belly. She almost fell off the treadmill, she was so rocked by this stranger. They ran side by side for twenty minutes more, and as soon as Rose finished her run, Simon stopped his machine so he could offer his help on the exercise machines. As they made a circuit of the weight training equipment, Rose and Simon kept up a saucy but easy conversation. Rose felt a powerful attraction to this gorgeous guy, and she had no objection to giving Simon her telephone number so they could help each other train for an upcoming marathon.

Rose had barely opened her front door when she heard the phone ringing. "I can't stop thinking about you," Simon said. "Can I come by?" *Yes!* Rose exulted to herself. *He feels it, too!* She got herself together enough to whisper casually, "Sure, why not?" Fifteen minutes later, Simon was there. They stared at each other, both glistening from their workout at the gym and the exercise program they were about to launch in Rose's bedroom. Rose knew this was destiny calling. She took Simon's hand and led him into the bedroom.

Two hours later, they were sharing a protein drink Rose had whipped up on the blender, and Simon was telling Rose about his Asian live-in girlfriend. Rose was thrown by this revelation, but she was still convinced that Simon and she were meant for each other and that Simon would eventually realize that he needed to be with a real sister. She continued to meet Simon for quickies in his car and invite him over for booty-knocking sessions for nearly eighteen months.

Rose admitted to me that she believed sex wasn't the only bond she had with Simon. "He told me that I was so exciting, he didn't have to look for other girls. That I was all he needed to relieve the boredom of his sex life with his girlfriend. I have to admit I got a charge from that; I felt proud. I even felt that I was sacrificing a real relationship for the moment because I was working for the cause—

returning a brother to the fold. I just knew he'd eventually wake up and realize I was the woman for him. In the meantime, I actually believed that I was doing Simon's girl a favor by keeping the number of his outside women down to one, not to mention helping out all my sisters out there by trying to win back a lost sheep."

Rose believed she was on an exalted mission, yet she felt empty every time Simon left her bed. She finally woke up to the folly of her sacrifice and broke it off, but she went on to form other star-crossed relationships with men who were either married or had girlfriends. Eventually, Rose couldn't deny her unhappiness any longer. She sought out therapy.

"I realize, now that I look back, that I settled for sex by convincing myself that I didn't want more," she told me. "I told myself I would eventually reap the rewards of my sacrifice. I tried to believe that everything was fine, that I didn't need any messy emotional involvement at the time—that I could wait until a man woke up and realized that he wanted me for life. But there was no real communication, and I could never count on any of these men to show up when they promised. They never took me out and showed me affection in public, and, to quote Nina Simone, I always slept alone. The real problem was my own emotional issues, that I believed sex on the run was all I deserved."

Being black and being a black woman does not mean you have to suffer or settle. As motivational speaker Tony Robbins states, "It is time to awaken the sleeping giant within." As men, women, singles, couples, and as a race, we must wake up from complacency and denial and recognize that we deserve better than we've been giving each other.

Now Is the Time

The great jazz saxophonist Charlie Parker once exclaimed, "Now is the time!" It's way past time for us to address inequities in education and the workplace, police brutality, and the factors that contribute to our higher risks for disease and death. Now is also the time to break out of complacency and denial and address the destructive ways in which we relate to each other.

In order to conquer CDS, we must first acknowledge that we are capable of doing better. If knowledge is power, then we must increase our knowledge so we can make a concerted effort to understand exactly how our PTSD destroys our relationships. We must wake up our community by collectively addressing this issue and its impact on us, through our educational and religious institutions, public forums, seminars, and books like this one that focus on our relationship issues. We must also be willing to offer honest opinions as professionals, neighbors, and friends—in a respectful and tactful manner—to those of us who are complacent or in denial. We must encourage our public figures, researchers, social scientists, doctors, psychologists, counselors, and religious leaders to openly address our relationship problems and the effects of our PTSD.

I lead relationship workshops and seminars because I believe venues that offer the opportunity for men and women of color to come together are vital and wonderful ways to share our intelligence, emotions, spirit, and information. These forums promote awareness and constructive strategies and advance our healing. These venues allow for face-to-face communication on key issues and the kind of structured experiences that bring us deeper understanding and a sense of community. Two or more heads are better than one, and many heads working toward the same goal can accomplish miracles.

Let's Pull Our Heads Out of the Sand!

Denial is a defense mechanism created by our egos to put blinders over our eyes and plugs in our ears so that we're unable to experience our lives as they truly are—without the fictional version we've concocted. When we're stuck in this trance of denial, we believe that what we think, feel, and see is the truth.

When we're in denial, we live inside the protective bubble of a self-created illusion that narrows our vision. Imagine being in a lush forest, teeming with all manner of trees, plants, animals, reptiles, and insects. Yet all you can see is a tiny patch of dead leaves. That rotting pile of vegetation fascinates you, so you pull out your camera and snap a photo. When you return from your trip, you show this photo to family and friends. "This is all I saw," you are saying. You never even noticed the varied spectrum of natural beauty that was around you.

Admittedly, we slip into denial, not to deny the beauty that surrounds us, but to protect ourselves from painful, far less attractive realities. Denial is so commonplace in our society that we are almost taught to look the other way, to point the finger and blame others for our problems. This self-delusion keeps us stuck on the belief that we're the saints and our partners or dates are the sinners. We are left angry, resentful, and, most of all, powerless to change the situation. We are left with the pile of rotted vegetation and cut off from the beauty of the rain forest.

How do we shake off the blinders of Complacency-Denial Syndrome so we can get down to the business of tackling the issues in our relationship styles?

We begin by pulling our heads out of the sand and looking around us so that we can make an objective, honest assessment of our relationship or dating patterns and determine whether or not complacency and denial have blinded us to the truth of those patterns and numbed us to their destructive effects. Yes, this is hard work, and waking up to reality can be as shocking as a dip in an icy pool on a steamy summer day. But it's good for you, an essential part of our quest for happier, healthier lives and more fulfilling relationships.

This chapter has already provided you with enough information to determine whether you are stuck to some extent in CDS. If anything you've read so far has raised a mental red flag, you probably identified a problematic aspect of your relationship style that's somewhat clouded by CDS. And if you've identified with any of the people whose stories I've recounted here, you may be in a position similar to theirs. If you still can't determine whether your vision has been obscured by CDS, try the following reality check:

This exercise helps you recognize the truth of your relationships. You do not have to score answers and add up the results. If you answer "yes" to one or more questions, you are experiencing some degree of CDS. That does not mean you are a failure or should be punished. These questions are designed to get you thinking. Your goal here is greater awareness—the first giant step toward positive change.

Reality Check for CDS: What Is the True State of Your Relationship?

1. Are you unhappy in your relationship or with your relationship style?
   Yes _____ No _____ If yes, list some reasons why: _____
   _____

2. Do you think your relationship or relationship style could use improvement?

Yes _____ No_____ If yes, list ways in which it could im-
prove:_____

_____

3. Do you feel you are overly forgiving of the negative or hurting behaviors of a partner or others?
Yes _____ No _____ If yes, list how: _____

_____

4. Do you believe that others, especially love partners, take advantage of your kindness?
Yes _____ No _____ If yes, list how: _____

_____

5. Do you believe that relationships by nature are supposed to
be difficult or painful?
Yes _____ No _____ If yes, list reasons why: _____

_____

6. Do you suspect that your partner has cheated or is cheating
on you?
Yes ___ No _____ If yes, list reasons why: _____

_____

7. Do you often find yourself feeling angry or sad, but you don't
really know why?
Yes _____ No ___ If yes, list the circumstances that make you
sad or angry. Be sure to include any connection to your relationship: _____

_____

8. Are you experiencing medical ailments that cannot be linked
to a physical cause?
Yes___ No___ If yes, describe the ailments: _____

_____

9. Do you believe that sex is not a vital part of a committed relationship?

Yes _____ No _____ If yes, list reasons why: _____

_____

10. Do you believe that anyone who expects his or her partner to be faithful is naive?

Yes _____ No _____ If yes, list reasons why: _____

_____

Again, if you answered "yes" to one or more of these questions, chances are that you are experiencing CDS. Of course, the more "yes" answers you have, the more serious and widespread are your complacency and/or denial. Check over those "yes" answers. They will be the catalyst that leads you to take the following action steps toward addressing, confronting, and eventually eliminating your CDS.

Action Steps Toward Eliminating CDS

- Every single day, either in the morning right after you wake up or before you go to bed, review your questionnaire. This is your daily reality check to remind you that you must continually work on confronting and resolving your CDS. This daily reminder prevents CDS from taking over your mind, so you are free to form more accurate perceptions about the state of your relationship. Think of the questionnaire as your daily relationship vitamin.

- As you look over the questionnaire each day, choose one question to which you answered "yes," and make a concerted effort to correct that negative behavior during the day. For example, if you answered, "yes" to "I am unhappy in my relationship," write out the specific reasons why. You might write out the following reasons:

"My husband is not intimate enough with me."

"My husband spends more time with his buddies than with me."

"My husband no longer takes me out on dates."

Formulate an action plan for that day that will correct that "yes" answer by improving your situation. Write these solutions down on the questionnaire. For example: "I will be less complacent about my husband's lack of sensitivity to me by doing the following:

On our way to work, I will ask my husband to hold my hand. I will ask my husband to kiss me in the morning and/or in the evening.

I will insist that my husband spend Friday night at home watching a video with me or taking me out."

- Incorporate these corrective actions into your daily review of the questionnaire, and you'll be more likely to implement these solutions on a regular basis.
- Go one step further by asking your partner to complete this questionnaire with you. Or you can each fill in your responses separately and then share the results. This way, you are addressing your problems and exploring possible solutions together. First, establish how you both contribute to CDS, and then brainstorm together for new, more productive relationship behaviors that will help both of you combat CDS every single day.
- In order to ensure that you and your partner address the CDS issues on a daily basis, each of you can sign a pledge—a simple agreement stating that you will both try to be more aware and attentive to any relationship problems that arise. Frame the

pledge and place it where you can easily read it every day. You can commit to tackling at least one issue per day, even if only for a few minutes.

- Depending on the severity of your CDS issues, try to make your daily explorations with your partner more fun and less confrontational. Go over the questionnaire and generate answers and healing behaviors while in bed together or while you're enjoying a nice breakfast or dinner.

- Practice zero tolerance when it comes to unacceptable behaviors from your spouse or partner. Stop being so forgiving. Stop looking the other way. Stop being so damn nice. Open your mouth and let your dissatisfaction be known. This is especially crucial when it comes to issues of domestic violence. Tell someone who can help. Protect yourself—the life you save may be your own.

- Don't be afraid to develop a new attitude about a long-standing problem. Just because you and your partner have let matters go on for so long doesn't mean you are too old to learn new tricks and develop healthier behaviors.

- If you are experiencing health problems unrelated to any physical causes, discuss with your doctor the possibility that the cause could be problems in your relationship patterns. In order to get the best treatment, you must explore the possible influence of any factor—physical or psychological.

- If you've gone through the questionnaire and suspect that your partner has been cheating, stop the music! Let him or her know this behavior will not be tolerated and that you must take immediate action, such as couples counseling. If your partner refuses to address the issue or continues to cheat while you're struggling to work out your problems together, it's time for hard decisions about what action you should take.

- If you still find yourself frequently angry, sad, or generally upset, redo the Reality Check Questionnaire to check whether these feelings are related to your relationship. If so, allow your discomfort to spur you into constructive action. Identify exactly what aspects of the relationship are creating these emotions and address them with your partner. The more action you take toward addressing the causes of your sadness or anger, the less likely it is that these emotions can overwhelm you.

- Explore individual counseling or marriage counseling. Even if you believe you have a good relationship, counseling can only improve your relationship. Even if you believe you've stripped away any traces of complacency or denial, you could be fooling yourself. Let's face it: no one is perfect. We could all use more insights into how to create happier lives.

- If you cannot afford counseling, don't have the time, or your area lacks this resource, invite a group of friends for coffee and a chat at least once a month, so you can discuss the issue of our PTSD and the behaviors it creates, including CDS. These groups are fantastic, because each participant both learns and teaches as members share their experiences and life lessons and give each other reality checks.

- Finally, once you have fully identified and eliminated your CDS behaviors, do not allow yourself to drift back into those old ways of functioning. The ability to evaluate your relationships with clarity and objectivity is a major strength. It equips you to make better choices and take charge of your life. It frees you to address whatever needs to be changed and to ensure that your relationship experiences become more healthy and loving.

CHAPTER THREE

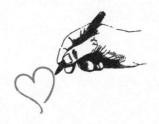

ENDING THE BLAME GAME AND TAKING RESPONSIBILITY

Once you've awakened from the slumber of your Complacency-Denial, the next step is to assume your share of the responsibility for your relationship woes.

Marilu's tumultuous six-year-long relationship was based entirely on blame. At forty-three years old, Marilu was still yelling about how everything was Jack's "fault." One of the first things she told me during her initial visit to my office was that Jack never washed a single dish—*ever*—that he never helped their son Luke with his homework, and, most of all, that his hot temper made their home an inferno. In fact, Marilu confided to me, "For the past two or so years, I've had to drink at least a six-pack of beer a day just to survive. The man is driving me to drink!"

To make sure that Marilu was looking at the entire picture and not just focusing on a narrow area of blame, I asked her to list the good things Jack had to offer as a husband and a father. It took her a month to come up with eight attributes, and some weeks she could only come up with one.

1. When he's not flying off the handle, Jack is affectionate to me and our child.

2. He's reliable.
3. Despite his frequent outbursts, he never goes beyond irritability and he never stays mad for long. Plus, he's always apologetic afterward.
4. He spends a lot of time playing sports with Luke on weekends and evenings.
5. He's a dedicated worker at his job.
6. He's generous with his family.
7. He is an avid carpenter who has made our home very comfortable.
8. He's got a great sense of humor.
9. Whenever we find the time to go out, we have lots of fun together.
10. We have many interests and hobbies in common.

As long as Marilu focused on Jack's quick temper, she was unable to see the entire picture. In fact, she blamed Jack for everything, including her own worsening alcohol problem.

Of course, abuse is never acceptable, and some relationships do need to end in order to complete themselves. But we tend to focus on what's not working or is unacceptable in a relationship, and it's far too easy to use blame as a way to justify our position in the relationship. We focus on the small picture—what the other person does wrong—all the while convincing ourselves that we're seeing the whole truth. But it's far better to be happy than to be right, so we must open up to the possibility that things aren't always what they seem, so we can make the necessary changes that will improve the situation.

It's never a case of "his fault" or "her fault": "She makes me hit her." "He makes me want to cheat." "The marriage turned me into an alcoholic." Both partners always share equal responsibility for their misery. It's funny how most people enjoy talking about themselves, but when it comes to why their relationships are mired in quarreling and other difficulties, the subject usually switches to a catalog of their partners' faults.

Like CDS, blame is a convenient defense mechanism. If CDS is about "hear no evil; see no evil," blame is about "I do no evil; it's all my partner's fault." Blame is yet another way to refuse the truth looming large right in front of us. In fact, CDS and blame often travel together. If we deny our pain and the truth of our circumstances, we're also refusing to take responsibility for our less than wise choices. It's far more convenient to blame the dismal results of our choices on the other party. When was the last time you remember anyone, including yourself, taking responsibility for negative outcomes in his or her life?

Blame: The Easy Way Out

Blame is the major obstacle that keeps people from taking responsibility for their actions, especially when those actions have a negative impact on the quality of their relationships. Yet taking responsibility for one's actions may be the most powerful way to heal relationships and turn them into success stories. Once you get past blaming your partner for every snag in your life together, you are able to challenge how you perceive that person. Once you overcome the convenient habit of blaming, you realize that you do not have to be a victim of negative relationships or any other undesirable circumstances in life.

You no longer have to be a victim, because overcoming a blaming attitude is empowering. Taking responsibility for your actions within your relationships means you acknowledge that you have choices. Choices give you control over your destiny! What a wonderful, exhilarating power responsibility can bring!

Ironically, whenever we blame others for our bad relationships, we believe we're protecting ourselves. Yet shifting the responsibility for our fate onto someone else means that we lose power over the situation. If everything is the other person's fault, then only that partner can change matters. After all, we've handed them all the control. Yet everyone knows it takes two people who assume responsibility for their own actions to bring about positive change, even in situations where one partner appears to be "the one at fault." The partner of "the one to blame" always has a choice: accept the situation as it is, change it, or leave.

How can we move past this troubling habit of casting blame elsewhere? Once we can be honest about what is really going on in our relationships or dating patterns, the next logical step is to assess whether we've been playing the blame game to escape responsibility for our choices.

Once we overcome the habit of blaming, we open ourselves further to challenging our perceptions of people and our relationships. Making necessary changes to get what you want becomes so much easier. In fact, the ability to take responsibility for your actions is one of the most powerful predictors for the success of your relationship.

Playing the Blame Game

We all know how the blame game plays out on the corporate level. When all is well for the corporation—production is high and profits even higher—who gets the credit? The boss. He or she is more than happy to explain how his or her heroic strategies led to the good times. When all is not well in Corpland, though, the boss tells another story. Who's to blame? Either lower-level workers or unfair, devious competition. The boss rarely looks to his or her own faulty management style as the cause.

In personal relationships, the blame game follows a similar pattern. When the relationship is bumpy, each side blames the other for the obstacles and rough spots. Some blamers even go outside the relationship to point a finger at The Man—the job, the landlord, the boss, or the racist society.

Blame is a way to escape our emotional tough spots, and we protect this escape route in several ways:

Operating in a Vacuum

It's easy to blame our partner when we refuse to communicate with him or her. If we operate within a vacuum, no one is there to refute our beliefs. Our reality becomes the sole reality, so we can twist and distort the facts of any situation in order to make our own beliefs, assertions, and behaviors seem more "right" and solid.

Chanson attended therapy sessions at my clinic because she wanted help in bailing out of her "horrible" marriage of four years. "Where is your husband?" I asked when she first came to my office. "He should be part of the sessions."

"Why should I bring him here?" Chanson wanted to know. "He's made my life a living hell. I'm here to figure out how to get out of this mess."

"Wouldn't it be fair to have him come here and see if the marriage can be repaired?" I asked.

"He's too screwed up," Chanson insisted. "He'll never change his ways, and it's his fault the marriage is so bad."

"How have you contributed to the relationship's problems?" I asked.

"I didn't and I don't," she said adamantly. "He is completely screwed up. He is at fault, and the marriage will never work."

Chanson refused to accept the possibility that she may have contributed to her dysfunctional marriage. She complained that her husband lacked ambition—he'd rather slave at a minimum-wage job than train in the evenings for a real career. Every time Chanson asked her husband to help her with their eighteen-month-old daughter or to do a few chores around the house, he complained that he was too tired. Yet on weekends, Yusef had plenty of energy to tinker with the vintage Mercedes Benz he kept in his cousin's garage. Chanson was also eager to have another child, a brother or sister for her darling Sylvie, but Yusef showed little to no interest in having sex. In fact, he was always glued to the TV screen when Chanson was ready for bed. After a few sessions focusing on Chanson's non-stop complaints, I finally persuaded her to bring her husband to my office.

Once both partners were present, Chanson was forced to listen to her husband's interpretation of their problems and confront his version of their life together.

"Chanson, this family thing was your idea, not mine," Yusef told her. "Had it been left up to me, we would have waited to have children until we'd saved more money and were in our own house." Yusef went on to reveal how overwhelmed he felt by the responsibility of a family, and that he even fantasized about running away. He just didn't know how he would ever earn enough to support them in the style he wanted, and this new pressure to have yet another child they couldn't afford was driving him crazy. He stayed up late at night, watching TV in the living room, to get a few moments' peace alone, and, yes, to avoid sex with Chanson. He was terrified that she would become pregnant again.

Chanson soon recognized that she had to accept 50 percent of the responsibility for their problems. Before counseling, Chanson was firmly entrenched in blaming that was enabled by operating within the vacuum of her own reality. Once Yusef entered the therapeutic process and Chanson heard how he felt and understood how she had contributed to their conflicts, she knew her marriage could be improved. But it would require hard work from both of them. Each partner would have to stop blaming and begin taking responsibility. It's easy to win a war when you are the only warrior, but if your goal is peace, you must allow the other party into the discussions.

Gender Stereotyping

Blaming is also facilitated by playing the gender card with lines like "all black men are dogs" or "black women just want a brother for his money."

Invoking gender stereotypes in order to deflect blame away from yourself is like calling on an entire army of your sex to back up your attack. Of course, you're blameless in the situation, because all black women know black men are dogs! Or, all black men know sisters just want a man for his money! Everyone says so!

Lynne had developed quite a reputation for loving and leaving men. Yes, the girlz are fully capable of hitting it and quitting it too! Yet Lynne proclaimed loudly and frequently to her friends and family that all she wanted in life was one good man.

One day, Lynne was out having lunch with her girlfriend Sylvia when she noticed a handsome dark-skinned man eyeing her from a nearby table. "Sylvia, tell me if I'm crazy. Check out that table to your right, with that tall, dark, and gorgeous piece of something. What do you see?"

"I see a very attractive brother checking out my best friend," Sylvia replied with a smile. "Why don't you go over there and say hi?"

"I don't think so!" Lynne replied.

An hour of eating and chitchat passed, and suddenly Lynne looked up to see the tall, dark stranger standing over their table, smiling.

"Hello ladies," he said. "I couldn't help but admire two beauties, and I had to come over and see if the one I'd been checking out was free. My name is Damien."

Sylvia got up hastily, mumbling that she had to visit the little girls' room, and Damien asked if he could sit down for a few moments.

"I think it would be fun getting to know you a little better," Damien told Lynne. "Here are two cards so you won't lose one. I'll be checking my e-mail every day until I hear from you. Have a lovely day. I'd stay longer, but I have to get to court. Also, say good-bye to Sylvia."

"I saw the entire episode," said Sylvia, as she slipped back into her seat. "I sure hope you e-mail him!"

Lynne waited two days to e-mail Damien, and he immediately asked her out to dinner that evening. During their date, Damien really seemed interested in her, but Lynne found it hard to believe that this blue-ribbon man was so fascinated with little ole forty-pounds-overweight her.

They saw each other constantly for nearly a month. "I'm falling in love with you," Damien told Lynne one night after they'd made love. "I've never felt this way about anyone. I've never met anyone like you. I think about you all the time, and you turn me on left, right, and center. Lisa is in shock that I'm in love with you."

Lisa? Lynne exclaimed to herself. What did Damien's paralegal have to do with it?

Lynne soon found out one day when she showed up a few moments early to meet Damien at his office. She ducked into the ladies' room to freshen up. While she was in a stall, she heard two women come in.

"What do you mean he's in love with her?" a woman's voice snapped. It was Lisa! "The woman is overweight, and Damien is going through a midlife crisis or something. What the hell does he see in her?"

"She's beautiful and she has class," said the other woman.

"She's a fat pig," exclaimed Lisa. "I'm going to have him back in bed tonight!"

"He's an honest man and you blew it, Lisa," said the other woman. "Damien will never trust you again. Plus, he told me he's in love with Lynne."

Lynne stayed in the stall until the click of their departing high heels died away, then crept out and checked the hallway. The coast was clear. She hadn't known that Damien used to see Lisa. To Lynne, that was a typical black-man move. What had she been thinking? Why had she fallen for his lines? He was a betrayer, just like all the other brothers she'd known. Even Sylvia, so happy with her faithful husband, was headed for a fall. It was just a matter of time.

Lynne ignored the other woman's testimony to Damien's love because she fixated on what she believed was evidence of his unfaithfulness. She headed back to her office and refused to take Damien's calls. As far as she was concerned, it was over.

Luckily, Lynne was in therapy with me at the time. When she related this incident to me, just as I've told it to you, I was able to point out how her stereotypical views of black men were obscuring her vision of who Damien was and exactly what he had and hadn't done. I argued that if she took every piece of evidence into account, the case came out decidedly in Damien's favor. Lynne was finally persuaded that she'd jumped the gun on her blame game by unfairly condemning Damien as just another worthless brother. She was able to open up to him and explain how she had felt. Damien understood and apologized for not telling her about his former affair with Lisa.

This crazy style of playing the blame game rears its ugly head frequently among same-sex posses that hang out at clubs and other public gathering spots and snicker to each other about the "opposition." Remember the gathering of sisters in Spike Lee's movie *Jungle Fever*? Every single relationship issue was automatically laid at the feet of the black man. The longer the session went on, the thicker the accusations flew—most based on tired, PTSD-induced stereotypes. The next chapter will dig deep to uproot these PTSD-associated stereotypes. For now, though, let's just imagine what would have happened if men had been invited to *Jungle Fever*'s male-bashing session. Or what would happen if females were invited into the men's locker room.

Perhaps those guests would offer their side of the story and bring a different, more complete and accurate reality to the party.

Again, my relationship seminars are popular because they provide that kind of opportunity for everyone to break out of the vacuums of their own minds and perceive each other as individuals instead of stereotypes. These seminars provide a welcome and much needed reality check for both sides of our gender wars. They give us a chance to stop blaming, start understanding, and finally assume our fair share of the responsibility for our relationship issues.

Automatic Anger and Temporary Relationship Insanity—TRI

We all know that anger can color our perception of any situation. Whenever we are consumed with anger or rage, we tend to lose our reason. We are so swept away by emotion that we find it difficult if not impossible to perceive others and the situation accurately.

Anger is a particularly significant cause of relationship difficulties within the black community. Black men and women have good reason to be angry. We're angry about our enslavement and about still being kicked in the butt every day by racist attitudes and institutions. We're also angry about the lack of nurturing relationships with each other.

Our anger may be justified, but it doesn't help us. Anger is a red cloud that obscures the clarity of our perceptions. Anger enables us to view situations in a distorted way so we can off-load our personal responsibility for our unhappy situations by blaming our partners— or any other convenient target.

Habitual anger in relationships can also lead to a condition I call Temporary Relationship Insanity, or TRI. We'll discuss TRI in depth in a later chapter, but for now it's important to recognize that TRI is an intensely negative level of blame that seriously warps our interpretations of a partner's behavior.

In my male therapy group, Santos bitterly accused his wife Josefina of deliberately making his life miserable. Santos and Josefina had been married for over eight years, but it seemed as if every action on her part, no matter how trivial, hit him with the force of an outrageous insult and provoked an explosion of his temper. She served his coffee cold. She refused to feed him dinner when he got home at night. She purposely ironed double creases into his pants.

She took too long in the bathroom. She had an annoying habit of asking him if she was getting too fat.

It seemed as if Santos's rage intensified with each weekly session, until Josefina was to blame for everything that went wrong in his miserable life. After repeated challenges by other group members, and a homework assignment in which Santos was asked to list Josefina's good qualities and then compare them to a list of her faults, Santos began to rethink his relationship. He began to check his own behavior and recognize that his tremendous anger colored his perception of Josefina's behavior to the point where he actually blamed her for deliberately breathing in a way to annoy him. In addition, his constant outbursts kept his wife on edge, so that her actions naturally became more strained and awkward.

Once feedback from other group members sank in, Santos acknowledged his anger and calmed down. Anger no longer clouded his interpretations of Josefina's behavior, and Santos became more rational and stopped casting blame. He recognized that the double creases in his pants appeared only when he and his wife were rushing to get dressed and his criticisms made her nervous. Meals weren't waiting for him because Santos himself had not asked for dinner to be ready, or Josefina knew he was going to eat before coming home. Josefina's breathing was loud because she suffered from a chronic sinus condition. Santos stopped blaming because he was finally able to take responsibility.

Following Advice from So-Called Friends and Caring Family

Blamers love to bolster their game with the slanted opinions of friends and family members. When everyone agrees with our view, we feel empowered to continue blaming our partner for all our problems. Support can be affirming, but if it's distorted and one-sided, that cheering squad is only promoting your misguided blame game.

Tenisha's favorite topic of conversation was her husband's latest bit of foolishness and his many failures as a mate. When she wasn't making fun of him, Tenisha was crying that he stayed out on Friday night with his boys, that he left sopping-wet towels and dirty underwear all over the bedroom, and that he'd sexed her the night before, then rolled off and proceeded to snore. Tenisha's girlfriends and family members were more than eager to support her in blaming her husband for all her relationship problems. Tenisha was justified to complain because her husband was sloppy, inconsiderate, and uncaring of her feelings. After all, she had no end of stories to back up her complaints.

At first, it even seemed to me that Tenisha was right. Yet as we explored their relationship more deeply, we discovered that all this endorsement of her every complaint was automatic and perhaps unjustified. As I pointed out to Tenisha, how can anyone be 100 percent right or 100 percent wrong in every single situation, especially when it comes to the give and take required by marriage?

Tenisha began wondering if her friends and family were being too hard on her husband, especially since they bad-mouthed him routinely, even when she hadn't asked them to. My suggestion was simple: lock out the opinions of your close friends and family members. If you need a reality check, get it from friends who are not as invested in backing you up or from family members known to be frank and objective. Of course, your first source of counsel should be an open, brave, and honest look into your own heart. And whenever you do speak with others, present the situation as evenhandedly as possible. Don't weigh your interpretation too heavily in your favor by making consistently negative statements about your partner. I suspected that Tenisha's cheering squad enabled her blaming because they had only heard Tenisha speak of her husband in a critical way.

Tenisha followed this plan with tremendous results. She asked her friends and family members to stop dogging her husband. Not only did she receive more balanced viewpoints from more objective people she consulted, but once she retired her cheering squad, Tenisha was better able to examine her own behaviors objectively.

Stopping the Blame and Taking Responsibility

If we are ever to come together in love, we must accept responsibility for our destructive relationship behaviors. We need to recognize that our beliefs determine our behaviors. If we operate from a negative mind-set, our perceptions of ourselves and others reflect that negativity. We naturally act from our skewed beliefs and perceptions, so our behaviors will be equally negative and flawed. No matter how evil, lazy, or even violent you believe your partner to be, I guarantee that you hold some responsibility for the state of the relationship!

Stopping the Blame

Now let's take a look at how to withdraw blame and accept responsibility so that you can develop new and more productive relationship behaviors:

Defuse your anger so your perceptions are more accurate

As I stated earlier, anger, especially habitual anger, warps your take on relationships and creates distorted, preconceived notions about a partner or potential partners. Anger is also the perfect fuel for blame. Together, blame and anger create a vicious cycle: we blame out of our anger, and the blame feeds our anger!

How can we defuse the anger and stop this vicious cycle?

Identify the true source of your anger

First, recognize that your anger may not be a reaction to a partner after all. It could stem from other, unrelated situations—even childhood experiences. Those early experiences often form the blueprint for how we perceive others and what kinds of adult relationships we create. Of course, our PTSD, the unresolved trauma of our history in America, is another major reason for the anger we often misattribute to the actions of our partners.

The best way to cool down is by discovering the true source of our anger. Once we pinpoint the source, our understanding helps anger dissipate. Sometimes therapy or another form of counseling helps accomplish this goal. You'll find that withdrawing blame for your anger from your partner improves your relationship almost automatically.

Tom spent every moment of his therapy sessions complaining about his wife. She was a terrible person, an awful cook, and lousy in the bedroom; and—though he didn't have a scrap of proof—Tom was certain his wife was having an affair. The very thought of this affair filled him with rage, so Tom spent every moment of his waking life consumed with anger. He was convinced his wife was entirely to blame for his anger and misery.

Tom discovered over the course of many months that he was actually angry with everyone. He underwent more intense therapy sessions before he realized that he had been an angry individual long before he met his wife. Somehow it had slipped his mind that he'd been diagnosed with an anger problem when he was in his teens. Once we finally began tackling the true origins of his anger, Tom began to stop blaming his wife, and he felt significantly calmer. Without that red haze clouding his vision, he was able to regard his wife more clearly, and he recognized that his suspicions about her affair were completely unfounded. Actively addressing the roots of his anger in his childhood improved Tom's marriage, as well as every other aspect of his life.

Fire the cheering squad

As we've already discussed, cheering squads are often formed on the basis of gender stereotyping. Cheering squads seem to support us, but they often impede our self-knowledge and growth. They also further alienate men and women. Guys versus gals is a loser's game. The girls gang up to form a sorority of bitter, broken hearts, and the guys become a fraternity of coldhearted players. These sisterly and brotherly orders prevent us from accepting our partners or potential partners as individuals and fellow human beings. Instead, we lump partners or potential partners with the coven of evil beeyotches or the posse of wu'thless men. Once we no longer consider each other as human beings, all restraints are off and blame flies freely.

Again, my tried and true antidotes to this destructive trend are relationship forums, where I maintain a balanced mix of men and women. Whenever we engage in exercises designed to clarify a particular relationship issue, I pair off men and women, one on one. Why? It's essential that participants learn to consider each of our issues from both the male and female points of view. Mixed gender pairing also breaks up the gangs, those gender-based cliques that fall so easily into the blame game.

If you need a shoulder to cry on or a clear mind to provide a reality check, try seeking out someone of the opposite sex. His or her insights could be enlightening, even stimulating.

Ask yourself: Why am I always getting involved in crash-and-burn relationships?

Troubles in relationships often reflect unfinished business from childhood that created unconscious needs. You could be trying to make up for the pain of your childhood. Perhaps you never knew your father, or he left when you were young, or he was present in the home but emotionally distant. Your mother may have been overly critical, too busy supporting her family, or too involved with boyfriends to provide the nurturing you needed. These experiences can leave you with an unsatisfied longing that drives you to seek out what psychology calls "corrective emotional experiences." In other words, as an adult you are magnetized by partners and situations that help you recreate your childhood scenario. You get stuck in trying to get from those familiar types of relationships the love and caring you never received as a child. Of course, these partners and situations are guaranteed not to deliver what you crave. As each situation fails, you are consumed by even stronger longings and greater pain.

Could that be your problem? Have you been seeking corrective emotional experiences through your relationships? If so, counseling is your best option for sorting out the childhood issues that lead you to repeatedly bang your head against the wall of doomed relationships. Counseling can help unload the baggage of the past that weighs down the present.

Check yourself daily

Advice from others is often helpful, but the best counsel comes from rigorous self-analysis performed with courageous and, if necessary, brutal honesty. Trust me, friends, it's the way to go. The most harmful lies are the ones we tell ourselves. You already know how easy it is to take the low road and blame someone else for your problems. You also know that easy route won't take you where you need to go—to love. The only way to get there is via the high road, which means turning inward to confront and analyze how you contribute to your relationship issues. This is a constant task for us all.

A written journal is a very powerful method of self-discovery. Journaling also fosters self-discipline. As you write down your thoughts and read them over later on, analyze and evaluate your thinking to determine if you've been refusing your share of the responsibility.

A special relationship journal will help you focus on difficult situations with your partner or dating situation. Every morning or evening, make a list of your ongoing relationship problems in your journal. Under each problem, create two columns. In the left-hand column, write the name of your partner or a potential partner. In the right-hand column, write your name.

Match each negative behavior you've described in your partner's column with a corresponding negative behavior of your own. Even if you believe you have no destructive behaviors to complement your partner's, rack your brain until you come up with one. I guarantee that once you discover and describe your behavior, you will recognize how you have contributed to the situation.

Here's an example of a journal entry I once made regarding my own marriage: "My wife is not a good housekeeper."

I wrote this one out of blame. I believed that since my wife is home all day while I'm out there trying to bring in the bacon, she should respect my efforts by being a better housewife. Here's what I wrote in the two columns about the situation:

Dr. Jeff's wife	Dr. Jeff
My wife is not a good housekeeper.	In the morning and evening, I throw my clothes on the floor, expecting her to pick them up.

She doesn't cook dinner often enough.	I am rarely home for dinner.
She never keeps the refrigerator stocked.	I refuse to accompany her to the market, yet I complain about her overspending.

And so it goes. You get the idea. Once my journal forced me to confront my own behaviors, I realized that my wife is not such a bad housekeeper after all!

Emerge from your vacuum and communicate

Once you've become a pro at the writing exercise I just laid out for you, you can graduate to doing the exercise with your partner. Self-analysis is important and worthwhile, but you also need to communicate. Make the exercise a couple's effort and create the list of negative behaviors together. The feedback you give each other provides keener insights into each of your behaviors, and working on the journal together is a great way to keep the lines of communication open. If you and your partner do this exercise together regularly, blaming behaviors from each side don't have a chance to take root.

Never blame in front of the kids

We can't forget that children model our actions. Parents are role models, good and bad. If our kids learn about the blame game by seeing us play it, they will grow up to be blamers too. We must avoid this war strategy, not only for ourselves but also for our children. A genuine adult knows to take responsibility for him or herself. If your children learn from you that every woe can be laid at someone else's feet, they can't grow into the men and women they need to be. Instead, they will take the easy way out and blame others for their problems, just like Mom or Dad. If you demonstrate how an adult takes responsibility, your children will reap the benefits in every other aspect of their lives.

Stop being a victim and start creating solutions

Once you've determined how you contribute to your dysfunctional relationship patterns, work on changing these behaviors, one behavior at a time, one day at a time. You won't become a perfect person overnight. The key is to begin acting on your new understanding. Accepting responsibility is a giant step toward more effective problem solving within your relationships, because you now understand which of your actions erode love, trust, and intimacy. However, all this doesn't happen by magic. Daily self-examination is hard, constant work, and you must commit to making changes. You will have to work through the complacency, denial, blame, and reluctance to take responsibility every single day. Defense mechanisms don't give up easily. But tools like the journals and lists I have given you will help highlight and clarify whatever you need to address and change. Gradually, you will come to see yourself less as a victim of circumstance or your partner and more as an empowered individual who is worthy of love and empowered to make choices that will improve his or her relationships.

Again, I can't stress enough the importance of the writing exercises. They are your best guides to increasing self-awareness and resolving relationship problems. Keep in mind that your actions create a ripple effect that extends beyond your individual happiness. Once your will to make positive changes is so firmly set in place that blaming stops and taking responsibility begins, your partner is likely to follow your example. If he or she can't follow, you may have to reevaluate the basis of the relationship altogether. Even if the relationship ends, you will not have failed. You will have cleared the way for a healthier love.

CHAPTER FOUR

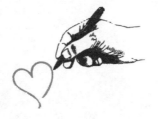

THE STEREOTYPE
TRAP

Complacency-Denial Syndrome and the blame game are just two of many leftover defensive mechanisms that no longer protect us. In the two preceding chapters, I provided you with strategies to help you substitute those worn-out PTSD behavior patterns with more constructive ways of relating to each other. One, these strategies will alert you to your true relationship issues. Two, they will show you how to assume responsibility for your choices. But we have more hurdles to overcome before we can create more stable, fulfilling relationships with each other.

Another set of worn-out behaviors stands in our way. These relationship behaviors were also inherited from the slave master, and we've also allowed them to continue distorting our perceptions of ourselves and each other. I'm talking about stereotypes, those distorted images about who we are as black people and what we're worth as human beings. I warn you: I'm going to get real here. We have to face up to the cold, hard truth: that we are sometimes guilty of playing into these stereotypes, and that's why these faulty images of ourselves are still holding us back. Stereotypes poison our self-esteem, our relationships, and our families.

Where Our Stereotypes Come From

Stereotypes are caricatures or exaggerated images created by one group in order to identify another group in a simplistic and negative way. Some typical examples of negative stereotyping include: Jewish people are cheap; Middle Eastern people are terrorists; Asians look alike; the Irish are drunks; and Italian Americans are tied to organized crime. Virtually every ethnic and racial group has been tagged with a laundry list of negative stereotypes. Of course, African Americans and black folks in general are no exception. Stereotypes about black people include that we're sexually well endowed and voracious, we recklessly father and mother children out of wedlock, live off welfare, are violent, and lack ambition and intellect. We all know these stereotypes are ridiculous. We are as varied and individual as everyone else, and most of us do not embody those stereotypical traits at all.

So what keeps these stereotypical views alive? Of course, most misguided and exaggerated notions about us are supported by the prejudice of nonblacks who perceive us through the degradation of negative stereotypes in order to maintain the illusion of their own superiority. After all, these stereotypes were created during slavery and colonialism in order to demean us and shake our confidence and thereby keep us down. If slavers and colonialists could drum it into our heads that we were inferior, we were more likely to passively accept our roles as slaves—beasts of burden and breeders.

Yet we can't pin the blame entirely on the master. We have done our part to promote and maintain these distorted images, and some of us have even created new mutations on the classic caricatures. How have we done this? By acting out stereotypical behaviors through our promiscuity, irresponsibility, dishonesty, and unfaithfulness, and by prejudging our own people through the distorting prism of stereotypes. Whenever we behave like irresponsible fathers or angry bitches, we feed into distorted notions about us. Likewise, whenever we dismiss *all* brothers as irresponsible fathers or *all* black women as angry bitches, we buy into the same distorted notions.

I'm not saying we shouldn't criticize our behavior in realistic and constructive ways. But it is patently false and unfair, for example, to dismiss all brothers as irresponsible and all sisters as angry.

We know that the stereotype of the irresponsible black father goes back to slavery, when fathers distanced themselves from their children in order to shield themselves from the pain of seeing those children sold and treated brutally. The stereotype of the overcompensating mama emerged as the conditions of slavery forced many sisters to soldier alone. Black women have been fathering and mothering their children from slavery days on down. These defensive behaviors helped us endure.

So why are we still acting out and reinforcing these distorted, one-dimensional images of ourselves? For example, why do few black men deny that they are studs, and many even boast of their sexual and physical prowess? Nothing's wrong with confidence in one's gifts, but if our sexual and athletic gifts are an excuse to dismiss our other abilities, other areas of human functioning, such as relationships, take a major hit. Our relationships become more fragile and volatile and less friendly, empathetic, and able to withstand the normal pitfalls encountered during the course of any relationship. We restrict our style of relating to each other to superficial, inauthentic encounters, because we bring only a tiny fraction of our full beings into the mix. Our relationships become a sham because we're not being real. Instead, we're hiding behind the mask of stereotypes that don't allow us to relate to each other as real people.

Let's dig deeper into some major stereotypes that are pinned on black people:

Male Stereotypes

John Shaft

The "John Shaft, he's a bad mutha" syndrome still runs rampant within our community and in the minds of American society at large. Of course, this bad mutha' was created by the slave master who needed a beast of burden to double as stud and slave-maker. Male slaves who went along with that program were valuable property and effective coppers, which won them a degree of status within and without the slave community. As an added bonus, their cold attitude protected these men from the pain of slavery. They were emotionally invulnerable to the master and—less fortunately—to their women and children. Again, this was the most effective way the black man could protect himself.

Sexual prowess is usually an effective means to achieve power because it plays off a basic human urge. Even if the slave didn't seduce the master's women, the slave knew the master feared that possibility. Along with that fear went envy of the male slave's sexuality. The male slave sensed that he possessed a valuable, even threatening commodity, so it isn't surprising that some black men became intoxicated with the heady feeling of being "so much man."

Again, sexuality is positive only when it is part of a full repertoire of other strengths. When a man brings a one-note sex samba to his postslavery relationships, he's off key.

Modern-day brothers who persist in acting out the Mandingo-bad-mutha-John-Shaft stereotype may consider themselves to be super ladies' men, but they are really presenting themselves as flat, pathetic caricatures.

Ken's womanizing didn't stop with his marriage to Glenda. He even cheated on her during their honeymoon. Glenda put up with it as long as she could, then filed for divorce and moved out of state.

I became acquainted with Ken after he became engaged to an acquaintance of mine, Lenora. Lenora had been warned about Ken's John Shaft ways by her close friend Annie, also a good friend of Glenda's. But Lenora couldn't resist. Her relationship with Ken was too passionate and romantic. Ken had a way of wrapping a woman up in a magical world, and he blamed his irregular calls and visits on his work as a salesman. "Being a salesman has its disadvantages," he told Lenora. "My life's not always my own. I have to meet clients at strange hours, whenever there's a chance for a sale. I know you'll understand. Glenda never could. She always nagged me about getting home on time."

Lenora didn't want to be like Glenda, so she was careful never to nag or demand explanations. One night when Ken failed to show up, she went to a movie alone and bumped into Annie. "Are you still seeing Ken?" Annie asked. "Yes, I love him," said Lenora. "Then I'm sorry for you," Annie replied gently. "If he was a woman, we'd call him a nymphomaniac. He only wanted Glenda for a safe haven, a mother figure to cook and clean and provide his home. He never stopped screwing around, and he's doing the same to you."

Lenora drove home, and Ken was there waiting for her—proof of his love. They married and went off to Jamaica for a golden honeymoon. On their last afternoon in Jamaica, they made love and Lenora fell asleep. When she woke up, Ken was gone. She wandered out to the beach that fronted their seaside cabin and spotted Ken in the distance, sitting very close to a laughing woman. She called to Ken, who explained that the woman was a potential sale and that he needed a little more time to close the deal. He told her to get ready for their flight the next day, then disappeared for two hours. Once they were home, Ken also explained the frequent female callers to their home and his sudden late-night departures as sale prospects. Whenever she asked if he got the account, he'd blow her off with a remark like "It's looking good, but I'll need another meeting."

One day, Lenora was sorting out the wash and emptied out the pockets of Ken's favorite pants. A package of condoms fell out. They were trying to get pregnant, so the condoms could only mean one thing: Ken was unfaithful. She confronted Ken who admitted he'd had women, "but they meant nothing to me." He promised to stop and be true to their marriage vows. Weeks went by, but Lenora still feared that Ken was cheating. One night she went through his briefcase and discovered a note from a woman that spelled out their relationship graphically and asked when they were getting together again.

Finally, Ken informed Lenora that he simply saw no reason to change. There were too many women out there in need of the services of a good man, and she was unreasonable to expect a man of his nature to sex only one woman. His love was for her alone, Ken said, and she'd have to find her security and happiness in knowing that. Lenora finally realized that her complacency had enabled her new husband's cheating ways. Since he was adamant about continuing his behavior, she left him, grateful that she hadn't become pregnant by this poor prospect for marriage and fatherhood.

Ken failed to realize that a true ladies' man is more than a sexual cliché. He offers a woman much more than a good time in bed.

Shaft types tend to view women in a one-dimensional way, as sex objects to be conquered and dominated. Those women who offer their hearts to John Shafts invariably wind up getting the shaft, figuratively and literally. The men may seem to be the winners, but they suffer as well. Their superficial style of relating to women forces them to hide their true feelings under the tough talk and callous behavior. In fact, these mackin' men are invariably unaware of their true emotional needs and the fears that block their love and vulnerability. These men get plenty of sex, but they miss out on the joys of true sharing and intimacy and the pleasures of gentle, deeply felt caresses. They never experience the happiness, security, and opportunities for personal growth that result from involvement in an honest, deep relationship.

Ritchie, a single man, also considered himself the ultimate ladies' man. He thought he was hip and cool—all that and a bag of spicy Bar-B-Q potato chips. He was a stockbroker, owned a deluxe crib on Manhattan's upscale Central Park West, and drove the latest Jaguar sports car. From the age of fifteen up to his present age of forty-five, he had conquered and bedded hundreds of women. Ritchie's belt couldn't hold all his notches. Every time he hit a club, he scored with the finest woman there. Ritchie was the envy of his male friends, single and married alike.

Ritchie's friends failed to recognize that not all was as it seemed. Ritchie had the game and the ladies, but his relationships never lasted. Yeah, Ritchie could rap to any female and take her home, but after a week or two at his time-share in the Bahamas, they were gone. In the beginning, his lady friends found Ritchie's credentials and suave style irresistible, but his superficial personality and lack of genuine emotion soon became a turnoff.

Ritchie didn't know what was missing, but he sensed something was wrong. As he grew older, he realized that he was not loved, and he became seriously depressed. At twenty-five, the mack role is fun, but playing sex machine wears thin by age forty-five.

Ritchie finally came to therapy. "I think I need help, Doc," he told me during his first visit. "I don't know why I can't find love or why none of my relationships ever last." His treatment involved figuring out where his Shaft persona originated and how he had maintained that false role through the adulation of his friends and the interest he still sparked in new women. Finally, Ritchie confronted the truth that he had to make changes in his thinking and behavior patterns. He also needed to address the realization that his sex-machine persona protected him from fears of intimacy and vulnerability. Ritchie had to revisit his childhood and early experiences with women to uncover the roots of those fears. Once the sources of his fears were exposed to the light of his mature understanding, Ritchie would be better able to risk an honest and straight relationship with a woman.

Where My Dogs At?

This stereotype spins off the John Shaft character. *Where my dogs at* may be the most common way our men destroy the possibility for genuine and intimate relationships. Again, like most of our dysfunctional behaviors, *where my dogs at* developed as a result of slavery and racism, when most male slaves couldn't afford to establish permanent liaisons with female slaves. Multiple sexual relationships helped them avoid attachments and the dangers associated with being a stable partner and father. It was safer to bond with other brothers, because these alliances might actually lighten the work burden and even increase the chance for escape.

Like other PTSD coping behaviors, *where my dogs at* has outlived its usefulness, yet some black males still believe their loyalty should be to their brothers, while they bed as many women as they can handle. Even some moms and dads boast about their male offspring's sportin' life. (Of course, the opposite goes for their daughters. Daughters who flirt freely and bounce from bed to bed are condemned as "loose" or "hoes.")

Where my dogs at is an even colder riff on the timeless male-bonding ritual we used to refer to as locker-room boasting, in which brothers gang up to support their view of females as tools for sex and procreation. The entertainment industry pushes this shameful stereotypical behavior. It rewards even baby-boy rappers for their junior-league mackin' by giving them such noms de guerre as Lil Romeo and Lil Bow Wow to signify that they'll eventually take over from older players like Snoop Dogg. All that doggish behavior is exalted in rhymes about sexual conquests and videos illustrating those lyrics with flocks of anonymous rump-shaking babes. To its credit, the movie branch of the entertainment industry is attempting to correct these negative stereotypes of manhood. Films like *The Wood*, *The Brothers*, and *The Best Man* promote the corrective notion that a real man does not prove his masculinity by sleeping around. A real man is faithful and responsible within his relationship.

Once you recognize that dogs band together for protection, *where my dogs at* behavior appears weak and ridiculous. Hangin' with the home boys in order to dog home girls is really about boosting sagging male egos through contests over who gets the most booty and makes the most comically derogatory statements about women. *Where my dogs at* is really about fear and the belief that strength in numbers will protect these men from that fear.

Where my dogs at behavior has also led many sisters to adopt a cynical view of brothers as faithless and "no good." If a sincere brother approaches a cynical sister, she's often too suspicious to trust him. She's labeled all black men as "irresponsible opportunists who are out to work the 'pum-pum' (to borrow another Caribbean term for female genitalia) for fun, a hot meal, a roof over their heads, or even a green card."

Even when couples somehow do get together, many marriages are destroyed because the man persists in *where my dogs at* behavior.

Convincing black men that they would be wise to shake an overattachment to their dogs is no easy chore. *Where my dogs at* behavior is addictive. These men can't believe they would be happier being best friends with their woman or dealing with one woman in an honest relationship. If they do attempt monogamy, they usually fall off the wagon at the first sign of trouble, because these men have difficulty sticking in long enough to work through problems and bring the relationship to a greater depth of intimacy.

Carl was late for his first marital counseling session, so his wife, Maria, used the time to pour out all her complaints about their relationship. Carl never spent time at home. He was always hanging out with his friends, partying as if he were single, and enjoying friendship with many different women. He was completely indiscreet, returning home with lipstick on his collar and reeking of perfume, and he constantly received calls from female friends. Maria suspected that he was dipping with at least a few of these friends, but Carl staunchly denied it.

When Carl finally made it into my office that evening, he didn't even bother with an excuse for his lateness. He had been with the "boys" and delayed paying his tab at a topless bar! Carl was not doing anything wrong. He and his boys were just having fun with each other and watching the girls. Boys will be boys, and that was completely normal, he informed me, even though he was spending less time with his wife and family than with his crew and other women. He saw nothing wrong with getting together with his posse to hit the bars and anywhere else they could party. Of course, Carl's dogs supported and encouraged Carl's inappropriate behavior, and when necessary, they also covered for him.

A few weeks into this couple's counseling sessions, Maria revealed that she'd caught Carl cheating. He'd told her one night that he was staying at one of the guys' home for a card session, but when she called there, Carl's friend said her husband had gone out for beer. Maria decided to check it out. She drove to the friend's home, but Carl wasn't there. Instead, she spotted his Jeep parked two blocks away, at a lady friend's house. Maria rang the bell and confronted them both at the woman's door—Carl in his underwear and the girlfriend in a flimsy bathrobe. The girl was shocked to learn that Carl had a wife, and she freely admitted to their affair. Carl had run out of excuses.

He was a tough case. An essential part of this couple's rehabilitation depended on Carl's recognition that his philandering behavior was not only juvenile, it was also destroying his marriage and family. Carl needed to grow up and recognize that the sporting life may be fun, but if he wanted a home life, he couldn't do whatever he wanted. Carl also needed to understand that certain people, places, and situations were trouble. He had to open himself to the possibility that if he channeled his sexual, physical, emotional, and spiritual energies into his relationship with his wife and children instead of wasting it on his dogs and other women, he might even enjoy greater happiness and fulfillment.

Once Carl realized how badly he'd been treating Maria and how hurt he would be if she had done the same to him, he understood that his behavior was actually sick. Admitting you're sick is the first step to recovery. Carl and Maria joined my couples group and began their journey toward a more meaningful relationship.

"Papa Was a Rolling Stone"

The Temptations' song lyric celebrates that "wherever [Papa] hung his hat was his home," but it also reflects yet another stereotype destroying the foundations of the black family. Again, this behavior originates in the black male slave's fear of becoming attached to one woman or family, and this behavior continues to persist—with a vengeance—long after slavery.

In fact, the "Papa Was a Rolling Stone" syndrome has worsened over the past several decades. It is the major reason why the black family is widely perceived as the stereotypical single-parent home headed up by a struggling, promiscuous, and uneducated sister who suffers from low self-esteem. We know that many of our black families are intact and nurturing, but we can't deny that too many black men fail to take care of their families. First of all, too many of us are fathering children without marrying their mothers, or siring babies with different women—and that includes married men who father children out of wedlock.

According to a new study by Steven Ruggles, a University of Minnesota history professor, from 1880 to 1960, the proportion of black children living with a single parent held steady at around 30 percent. During the same period, the proportion of white children living with one parent stayed at about 10 percent. In recent years, those figures have climbed—to 63 percent for black children and 19 percent for white.

Again, many black families are intact, and many black men take care of their babies. If we accuse all black men of being rolling stones, we sink to viewing each other as stereotypes. At the same time, though, we have to admit that too many brothers perpetuate the stereotype by living it out.

Just for the sake of argument, let's throw out some well-known names of men who should know better. Among them are Yankee Slugger David Justice, who is being sued for child support; P Diddy, who recently settled out of court with his former girlfriend for child-support payments; and the very married Reverend Jesse Jackson, who was threatened with civil action for increased child support by his former mistress. Of course, plenty of white men have children out of wedlock, but white males are not universally condemned as irresponsible fathers. Some are even viewed as "independent, free spirits." Yes, that's unfair, but as black people, we face too many challenges within this society to afford this behavior. Let's face it: some brothers believe it's perfectly fine to drop seed and keep on moving. They're even proud, as if having babies makes them more of a man, and they ignore the impact of their thoughtless behavior. Not only do the mothers feel abandoned and overwhelmed by the dual role of mother and father, but the children also suffer greatly. These children often fantasize about having a mother and father in the home and feel lost, abandoned, and worthless: "I wasn't good enough for Daddy to stay with me." These children often act out their lack of self-worth through behavior problems at home and in school. Statistics show that most people in prison were raised without the physical presence and guidance of fathers or father figures.

Susan became pregnant with her boyfriend David's child just as his family was hit by crisis. His father left his mother for a younger woman, and his mother was distraught. When Susan began spotting and had to stay in bed for several weeks, David chafed under the weight of the demands made on him by both his girlfriend and his mother. After a few weeks, David exploded when Susan insisted one more time that he marry her, as if that would ensure the safety of his unborn child. He stormed out of her apartment and never showed up again.

Susan gave birth to a little girl she named Tammy. By then, David was missing in action, and Susan was too angry to pursue her daughter's errant father.

I met Tammy fifteen years later, when she walked through the doors of one of my clinics, a teenaged single mom with two convictions for shoplifting. I can say with certainty that Tammy's premature motherhood and problems with the law were rooted in her profound sense of abandonment. Raised by an embittered single mom who had nothing but dismissive, curt comments regarding Tammy's father, and burdened by the deep-seated belief that her father would have stayed if she and her mother were more lovable, Tammy suffered from a seriously low sense of her worth. Without the unconditional love of a father, she settled for sex and early motherhood—a child who would love her—and didn't even believe she deserved a good education and a promising career.

These tragic situations fuel the tensions between our men and women. Single moms are angry and sad because their children's father is either not with them or fails to take care of their kids. The children are trapped in this dynamic, especially if the parents make negative comments about each other in the children's presence. Exposure to all this anger and resentment causes children great psychological distress and cripples their ability to grow into healthy, loving adults who are capable of establishing and nurturing their own long-term relationships.

This is how negative behaviors become a legacy that's handed down through the generations. Many absent or irresponsible fathers were raised without their own fathers. Despite the pain it caused them, these men came to accept their fatherless condition as the norm and to behave the same way. These men's bad behavior also expresses the unresolved anger they still carry from their fatherless childhoods, and they express their condition by being ineffective fathers themselves. Fatherless daughters often become women who also accept single parenthood as their expected lot.

Juan was a patient trapped in this generational pattern. His father lived in the same neighborhood where Juan grew up, but he'd never acknowledged Juan legally and refused to give him his last name. Juan's mother was his sole parent. By the time Juan fathered a child out of wedlock with his steady girlfriend, Beverly, he was already the father of two other children by two different women. Juan had begged Beverly to have their baby and promised to marry her as soon as his finances came together. After the birth of the baby, though, Juan did not follow through on his promise, even though he loved his girlfriend. Hurt and angry, Beverly kept the baby away from Juan. She finally relented, but now Juan refused to see his baby out of spite. Another child was destined to grow up with an angry mother and without his black father.

After months of therapy, Juan worked through much of his anger over growing up fatherless and recognized that he'd been taking out his pain on his own kids and their moms. In fact, changing the script of this generational legacy was his best chance for healing his own pain. He could not cause his children to suffer his own fate any longer. Juan admitted his responsibility to his children financially, physically, and emotionally, and reconciled with all three moms. Today Juan is married with two children at home, and his three kids out of wedlock spend every weekend with his family.

Female Stereotypes

Our women suffered equally if not more than our men during slavery. Female coping behaviors that once helped our women endure have also solidified into stereotypes that are alive and well today, long after they've outgrown their usefulness. These include "The Breeder," "Overcompensation," "No Money, No Honey," and "Punany Power."

Some female coping behaviors that evolved into stereotypes also began as defenses against the master's cruelty, but other behaviors developed to protect black women from their own men's hurtful and demeaning treatment. This is why many female stereotypes take the form of flipping the script on shoddy male behavior. These defensive coping strategies may seem to ease women's pain and anger, but over the long term, living out these stereotypes gets us nowhere.

Let's take a look at some common stereotypes sisters have developed:

The Self-Sacrificing, Overworked, Overcompensating Mama

No one can be faulted for being hardworking, responsible, and self-sacrificing. But if you view yourself as a martyr who has to take care of everything—especially because your man is useless—responsibility becomes a hell of a burden and exerts a powerfully negative effect on your relationships.

Let's examine how this behavior evolved. During slave days, slave women were often forced to sleep with the master as well as with various slave men, in addition to laboring in the fields or the big house. Female slaves were also forced to cope with male slaves' defensive, dysfunctional behaviors. The conditions of slavery forced many black women to become the sole stable force within the black community—even the community at large. Black women acted as caretaker for both the master's family and her own. In many other cultures, the matriarch is the backbone of the family, but that's particularly true within the black community. Our PTSD has ensured that too many black mothers still shoulder this overwhelming role of mammy or supermom.

Women who fulfill the stereotype of supermom on a full-time basis are so stressed that they often develop physical disorders. The federal government's publication "Changing America: Indicators of Social and Economic Well-Being by Race and Hispanic Origin" reports that black women in this country are three times more likely to develop cervical cancer than white women. Black women's death rate from pregnancy-related illness is four times greater than white women. Black women are also twice as likely to develop uterine fibroids.

Of course, the supermom role also has a destructive effect on black women's relationships with men.

Many women of color no longer trust in the competence of their men and truly believe that they can do better for themselves. These women are convinced they don't need men, except perhaps for physical pleasure or to carry heavy bags. Of course, any arrangement based exclusively on sex is doomed, and many women who take care of everything on their own are perceived as overbearing, controlling, and even castrating.

Overcompensating women can be guilty as charged. If you are accustomed to control, it's difficult to hand over the reins or even share the responsibilities of maintaining a relationship and running a household. Men in relationships with overcompensating women often wind up rebelling, and the relationships suffer. Children involved in these relationships grow up believing that women are omnipotent out of necessity and men are lazy and shiftless by nature. Boys believe they are expected to be irresponsible, and girls grow up expecting men to fail them.

Jakisa was a prime example of an overcompensating sister. Her mother taught her by example that black women had to be superwomen who work for themselves, their families, and their men.

Jakisa's father, Harry, had been struck with a horrible illness not long after Jakisa's baby brother, Brian, was born. For nine years, Jakisa's mother took over the entire responsibility for the household, waking up at 5 A.M. every day to bathe, dress, and feed her children, then take two buses to drop them off for the day at her mother's. From there, Jakisa's mom took a train to her job as housekeeper for a family in the suburbs. She rarely made it back home before 8 P.M.

Looking back, Jakisa never remembered her mother smiling. It was clear that life was an ordeal for her mother, and Jakisa, Brian, and their father were the reasons for her burden. Yet Harry had wanted to study computer programming at home, and he begged his wife to allow him to invest their little nest egg in a course and a computer. That way, he'd be able to earn a living from home and ease her burden. She refused, yet she continued to complain about being stressed and overworked. Finally, Jakisa's father informed her mother that he was leaving, that the stress of living with her was too much for him to be able to recover from his illness. Shortly thereafter, he moved out and disappeared from their lives.

Jakisa's mother was dumbfounded by her husband's abandonment—after all her sacrifices! And she never missed an opportunity to pass down her bitter lesson of betrayal to her daughter. Men were no-good, faithless dogs, she'd tell Jakisa. She only had to look at her father's example to prove her point.

Jakisa never considered the possibility that her mother had contributed to her marital woes by emasculating her husband, by blocking his attempts to find work he could do despite his illness, and by flooding him with a barrage of criticism and complaints. When Jakisa grew up and began having relationships of her own, she assumed that she had to do all the work, that men had to be led and couldn't be trusted to act right on their own. Fueled by images of her exhausted mother traveling back and forth from their home to the suburbs to clean and cook for someone else's family for a minimum wage, Jakisa became fiercely ambitious. She put herself through college by working as an office temp, then went to law school while working as a paralegal. Jakisa passed her bar exam on the first try and went to work for a prestigious law firm in her city.

Yet Jakisa consistently sought out relationships with men who were far less ambitious and hardworking. In fact, one man was a marijuana dealer. Almost in spite of herself, Jakisa finally met her match in Carter, when they opposed each other in a divorce case. After the case was over, Carter called Jakisa to ask if he could see her that weekend. Jakisa was attracted to Carter and she respected the thoughtful way in which he approached his work. She knew this was the kind of man she should date, yet something was holding her back. She just couldn't believe any good could come out of seeing Carter. Yet there was no good reason for turning him down, so they began going out together. After a few weeks, Jakisa realized that she was afraid and her fears could jeopardize this promising relationship.

She'd known nothing but a series of failed relationships with the weak men in her past, and she decided that this pattern was disturbing enough to seek help through therapy. She told me that she could not figure out why her relationships never lasted beyond a few months and the men always wound up resentful. Jakisa joined one of my coed groups, where she constantly complained about how much she sacrificed for her men. She bought them clothes so they would look more professional when they were in public and cleaned their apartments to help them organize. She failed to realize that all this "help" was actually her way of taking control. Carter didn't need her help, so she was at a loss about where the relationship was going. In fact, she admitted, she felt like a fish out of water, and that terrified her.

During a mixed-gender group session, a brother pointed out to Jakisa that in the past she'd acted like an overcontrolling, overresponsible mama who believes all men are too incompetent and irresponsible to do without her help. Carter was obviously a different type from her previous men, and her fears were based on her inability to take him over. Jakisa struggled to absorb that feedback, but she finally realized that she had to build trust in the competence of men, specifically in Carter. She also had to relinquish her belief that the only safe relationship was one she controlled. She began to view her relationship with Carter—and any other man she might date—as a fifty-fifty proposition.

The High-Flossing, Mercenary Babe

More and more young women are buying into the classic "no money, no honey" persona: "If you want my love, show me the money. It ain't about nothin' but the rent." This female stereotype is a mirror image of the John Shaft and *where my dogs at* personae: "If the guys exploit and use us for the pum-pum, they'll have to pay for it." Payment can be an expensive dinner, a new dress, or a check for the light bill. Whatever form the payment takes is not as important as the satisfaction of knowing the brother has paid. You may believe nothing's wrong with this line of reasoning, but it is fundamentally flawed.

The main flaw is that not all brothers play games and cheat, so good guys suffer for the sins of the bad. Another flaw is that whenever a woman places a price tag on her love, she cheapens its value. Men view these women as little more than high-priced call girls. A money-for-honey relationship is a business transaction, not a human interaction. Let's face it: money-for-honeys are regarded by both genders as tacky and lacking class.

Janie was the epitome of the high-flossing, money-for-honey woman. She had expensive tastes and couldn't be bothered to hide it. Janie firmly believed that if she put other people's needs before her own, they'd walk all over her, and that would bring more pain than she could handle. She'd grown up with a mother who struggled to raise her and her sister. After her mother died of diabetes and a heart attack at age fifty-three, Janie vowed she'd never work that hard for nothing. All her mother's hard work had worn her down and made her old before her time. Life would not take advantage of Janie. She would take advantage of life.

Janie's sister tried to warn her about her dangerous obsession with money and material goods.

"Girl, you need to change your ways," she told Janie. "You need to look for love. Life's too short for spending it alone. You need to find a good man and give him a chance." But Janie refused to listen. "What good is love?" she asked her sister rhetorically. "All it brings you is hurt and pain. Before you know it, your man is laid up somewhere else with some ho' and you're crying in the dark, like Mama."

Janie's girl conversation focused on one subject only: hunting the big game, men with money. She spent all the money from her job on Gucci shades, Prada bags, and the sexy little designer outfits she wore when she and her girls hit the upscale after-work clubs. Her friends were also interested in successful men, but these women were successful themselves and naturally sought out compatible mates. Janie was interested in money only. If a man wanted her, it would cost.

When she met Omar, an older man in his early forties who'd never been married and had only one child who lived with her mother, Janie believed she'd hit the jackpot. Omar owned a local chain of appliance stores and lived in a large mansion on a hill overlooking their small Southern city. They began dating, and it wasn't long before it was evident that Omar was falling in love. He took Janie to expensive restaurants and bought her gifts of gold bracelets and necklaces. All Janie cared about was what she could get out of the deal. She wanted her rent taken care of and her car note paid.

The first time they made love, Janie put everything she had into her performance. When they finished, Janie jumped up, put on her robe and asked Omar to leave. He was stunned, until Janie accused him of just wanting her for sex. When he protested that he'd do anything to prove he wanted her in his life, Janie pretended to turn sad and forlorn. She needed help with her rent and bills, she admitted, and she hadn't told him before because she didn't want to burden him with her problems. Omar was more than happy to tell Janie that her worries were over.

Janie had played Omar, but she justified her act to her girlfriends by saying that men always took so much from women. Why should she knock herself out working, then go home to a man who wouldn't even meet her halfway? Besides, Omar was nothing but an old-ass man trying to get with some young coochie.

Janie managed to work Omar for several months before he spied her at the mall, giving out her telephone number to a young man. "I can pay someone to give me the loving you give," he told Janie before he walked out and slammed the door. "After all, you carry yourself like a whore anyway!" Janie figured her only mistake was in being caught out. She continued her sugar-daddy game, looking for men who would take care of her and make sure she lived happily ever after.

Several of Janie's girlfriends did wind up marrying men of means and enjoying successful marriages based on compatibility and love. Janie is still out there. Over the years, her approach has hardened and grown obvious, so Janie now attracts a lower-quality man, the kind of guy who sees through her but doesn't care. This man is more than happy to buy the honey and leave once he's got his money's worth.

The Breeder

We already know that the breeder is the flip version of the Buck, that she fulfills a slavery-rooted stereotype that dictates the black woman's job on earth is to produce children. Sadly, some contemporary breeders continue to define their sexuality and worth by their ability to churn out children, often in order to express their love for a man and trap him—a ploy that's rarely effective. The breeder places little value on her other attributes, such as intelligence. Breeders are easy to spot, so men usually stick around for a brief period, then cut and run.

By age thirty, Selena had seven children and no husband. She had loved each of her babies' fathers, but she never managed to persuade a single one to tie the knot. When she met Xavier on line at the supermarket, she felt she'd finally found true love. Xavier was shockingly beautiful. To Selena, he looked just as if he'd stepped out of the pages of a body-building magazine. He told her that he taught Latin dancing at a local dance school, so Selena made sure to pay him a visit at the dance school the first chance she got. It wasn't easy getting out of the house with seven children at home, but Selena traded baby-sitting with a neighbor in her apartment building and dropped by for a beginner's class one evening and to check out Xavier's moves. Xavier seemed delighted to see her and paid more attention to her than to the other students. At one point, they were glued together, eyes boring into each other's souls while executing a move Xavier had just taught Selena. He pressed even closer to whisper huskily in her ear, "You are so sexy. I have to see you tonight." Then he withdrew, smiled, and gave her a soft peck on the cheek before he moved on to another student. Selena felt like a woman again. It had been too long since a man had whispered sweet nothings in her ear, especially a man as hot as Xavier. She slipped him her address as she left the class. An hour later, he was in her bedroom and Selena was trying in vain to stifle her screams of joy as he made love to her. A month later, Selena was pregnant with her eighth child, and Xavier was doing the tango with some other student in some other town. With each child she produced to win a husband,

Selena's chances of getting married to a good man had actually decreased even further. Let's face it: it's a rare man who's willing to marry the mother of many children fathered by several baby daddies. After much counseling in my office and visits to a family planning clinic, Selena had her tubes tied and was no longer able to bear children to bolster her self-esteem. Therapy helped Selena focus on exploring new ways to cultivate a sense of self-worth and on raising her children, instead of wasting her time trying to "trap" a man.

The Perpetually Enraged Black Woman

The conditions of slavery would make anyone holler. Releasing anger can relieve its pressure and stave off depression, but a chronic state of anger eventually wears you down because the causes for that anger have not been resolved. Though much of our anger originates in rage at the master for his monstrous acts, many female slaves also simmered with unconscious resentment toward their men for failing to protect them. After slavery ended, that resentment increased as white society continued to treat black women as third-class citizens and the black man continued to withhold his emotional intimacy. As a result, many of our women are perpetually enraged and attacking the guilty and innocent alike. No matter what a man does or says or how loving he tries to be, an angry woman bombards him with her rage in return. In fact, the woman usually lets it fly on any male, whether it's a fellow bus passenger, a service provider at the post office, or a stranger checking her out on the street. The anger can be so consuming that these women are incapable of establishing any kind of relationship with a man.

Stereotypical battling black women have few clues as to why their relationships fail or why they can't meet a man, because they are unaware that they're trapped in a vicious cycle. Their anger turns men off, yet each rejection causes these women's rage to escalate.

Marsha was angry with her children, her boss, and her husband; and, after starting therapy, she was even angry with me. Of course, everyone was to blame for her anger but herself. Her kids were not doing well in school, she wasn't making enough money, her boss treated her like a slave, and I refused to agree with her on every point. Most of all, though, Marsha was angry with her husband, Ben, for not giving her the love she deserved. Marsha was so furious, that she couldn't even express her feelings to him without shouting. Eventually, I asked her to bring her husband to a therapy session.

When Marsha confronted him during the session about not making love to her often enough, Ben finally yelled back that he wanted to love her, but her anger scared him off. He described their marriage as a long, tense walk over eggshells and admitted that he was too afraid to broach any subjects with her because, at the first sign of trouble, she invariably began to rant and scream. Marsha's first instinct was to defend herself by attacking her husband. But I wouldn't allow her to go off on a rant. I asked Marsha to consider the possibility that some of her behavior patterns were making it difficult for Ben to love her. The three of us went over his complaints to untangle the specific words and deeds that were building the emotional wall that separated Ben from Marsha.

One pattern that Ben found especially infuriating and demoralizing was Marsha's constant reminders that he was from the "wrong side of the tracks." Ben and Marsha had met one day when Marsha was walking home from high school. Ben was with two other boys who stopped Marsha and a girlfriend. One of the boys had gotten nasty and grabbed Marsha's hair when she tried to walk off. Ben had defended Marsha and ordered the other boy to let her go. She ran off, dropping her schoolbooks. Ben scooped them up and caught up with her to return them. He apologized for his friend's behavior and told Marsha he wouldn't be hanging out with that boy anymore. They were together ever since. Ben was three years older, a high school dropout, and Marsha would be a college student the following September. Yet they stayed in touch and married soon after Marsha graduated with a degree in elementary education. In the meantime, Ben had gone for his GED and trained on computers while Marsha was away at college. By the time she returned, he was earning a good living as a computer repairman. But Marsha never failed to tie her criticisms of Ben to his humble beginnings, and Ben's resentment over these reminders that he was from the wrong side of the tracks had reached the boiling point.

This revelation opened Marsha's eyes. The two of them continued to talk in counseling sessions and at home, and Marsha acquired some anger management skills. Finally, she began defusing her anger and learning how to reach out to her husband and others in more constructive ways.

Prejudging Through the Distortions of Stereotypes

Living out worn-out stereotypical patterns is only one part of the problem. The stereotype trap also includes the prejudgments we inflict on each other. Like Marsha, some of us have bought into these degrading images of ourselves to the extent that we hold the same low expectations of each other. Identifying with the aggressor is a common psychological fallout from oppression. When we are forced to accept degrading treatment over a lengthy period of time, we come to believe that we deserve it.

Viewing our significant other or a potential mate through the distortion of a stereotype, without offering that person a chance to show who he or she really is, can be as destructive as acting out a stereotype. Our expectations are so inflexible that the person usually winds up conforming to that negative prejudgment. Restricting people to stereotypes means we give in to our pessimism and suspicion. We convince ourselves that the individual is incapable of breaking out of the mold and displaying unique, sophisticated, and versatile behaviors. Trapped in our prejudiced mind-set, we are incapable of approaching our partner or potential mate as a friend. That person becomes the enemy, our opponent in this crazy war.

Even if a potential mate or partner engages in stereotypical behaviors, we must try to look deeper to discover his or her true self so we can discover more genuine ways of relating.

Shantella decided to seek psychotherapy after she was devastated by a broken engagement. Shantella had coasted through breakups in the past, but this one laid her lower than she'd ever believed possible. The problems had started when she just couldn't convince herself to marry Antoine, even though he had asked her twice. Shantella was convinced Antoine was incapable of committing to marriage. At forty-seven, Antoine was six years older than Shantella. But he was an attorney with a track record that testified to his appeal to the opposite sex.

Every time Antoine showed up at Shantella's office to take her to lunch or pick her up after work, she'd hear different women talking about Antoine and how they couldn't take their eyes off him. She had to bite her lip to keep from saying anything, but their remarks—always made in jest—made her nervous. Her friends didn't help either; they were more than happy to dig up information about the lengthy list of girlfriends he'd dogged in the past.

Antoine couldn't convince Shantella that he'd had enough of

the game. He'd hung up his cleats. He was through running and wanted to settle into marriage and raise a family. Shantella wasn't having it. At first, she was happy to be engaged, but every time Antoine tried to set the date, she got cold feet. He was too success-ful and good-looking, plus he was a black man, and she just knew sis-ters were on him like white on rice. With all that feline pressure, how long would it take for Antoine to cave in?

Shantella didn't realize until it was too late that Antoine had been faithful to their relationship. She'd received no sign that he wasn't true, but she persisted in her stereotypical view that all men are dogs, especially the "quality guys." Antoine was a good guy, but her constant accusations finally wore him down, and he broke off the engagement. Shantella had won the love of a wonderful man, and then she lost it because she insisted on judging Antoine as a John Shaft. Antoine wound up married to Shantella's so-called best friend, Shirley, a member of the female cheering squad that was con-stantly shouting in Shantella's ear that black men can't be faithful!

Fortunately, therapy helped Shantella learn how to approach men as individuals, and she's now happily married to another good man.

Let me share some of the advice I gave Shantella and my other patients for breaking out of the stereotype trap:

Action Steps for Breaking Out of the Stereotype Trap

Breaking away from stereotypical behaviors and judgments is not that difficult. All it requires are a few simple steps I describe as "stereotype smashers."

Step 1: Determining How We Live in or Perceive Stereotypes

We've already touched on my observation that many of us act out some form of stereotypical behavior. Of course, some of us inhabit these false roles more fully than others. As with all our PTSD behaviors, we are often unaware or in denial of what we believe and do to promote this negativity. In other words, Complacency-Denial Syndrome can blind you to where you stand on the stereotype issue and what negative effects stereotypes may be exerting on your relationships.

So, the first step toward escaping the stereotype trap is to determine whether complacency or denial plays a part in your behavior or your judgment of others. Read through the descriptions of stereotypical behaviors in this chapter once again. Where do you fit? You may be acting out one stereotypical character to some extent, or you may be spreading out a little, rather like choosing one stereotype from column A and two from Column B. For example, outside the home, you could be the high-flossing mercenary babe, but once you shut your front door, you snap into the overly-responsible-mama mode. You could be lumping all men under the John Shaft stereotype, or mixing it up and viewing them through the distorting filter of several negative images at once.

Let there be no shame in your game. No one is peeping over your shoulder as you read. Stay open to a thorough and honest examination of how stereotypes may be influencing your relationships. Once you know what you've been doing, you stand a much better chance of learning to substitute this behavior with a more effective approach to your relationships.

Step 2: The Stereotype Smasher Questionnaire

The following Stereotype Smasher Questionnaire will help you pinpoint more precisely how stereotypes influence your relationship behaviors. Be ruthlessly honest: your total of "yes" answers is not as important as the insights those answers will provide.

The Women's Questionnaire

1. Do you believe that your relationship behaviors or perceptions need no improvement?
   Yes __ No __

2. Do you believe having babies is the best way to keep a man?
   Yes __ No __

3. Do you believe that a man should give up his money for your honey?
   Yes __ No __

4. Have you had children out of wedlock?
   Yes __ No __

5. Do you believe you can never depend on a man?
   Yes __ No __

6. Do you often find yourself angry or reacting in an angry manner, especially within relationships?
   Yes __ No __

7. Do you believe all men are dogs?
   Yes __ No __

8. Do you believe men cannot be faithful?
   Yes __ No __

9. Do you believe most black men are irresponsible fathers?
   Yes__ No __

10. Do you believe black men are the enemy?
    Yes __ No __

The Men's Questionnaire

1. Do you believe your relationship behaviors or perceptions of the opposite sex need no improvement?
Yes __ No __

2. Do you believe your behavior is no different from that of other committed men, and therefore, hanging out with your male buddies all the time is okay?
Yes __ No __

3. Do you feel less guilty about acting single when you are with your buddies?
Yes __ No __

4. Have you had children out of wedlock?
Yes __ No __

5. If so, are you a responsible father?
Yes __ No __

6. Do you believe married men are entitled to a fling or two or three or more?
Yes __ No __

7. Do you believe black women are the enemy?
Yes __ No __

8. Do you believe sisters only want a man for his money?
Yes __ No __

9. Do you believe most black women are angry and difficult?
Yes __ No __

10. Do you believe most black women try to trap brothers by having children?
Yes __ No __

If you answered "yes" to one or more of these questions, you need to consider the possibility that you either behave in stereotypical ways or perceive others through limiting stereotypical images.

Now that we've raised awareness, let's move on to the next stage of stereotype smashing—taking action:

Step 3

Friends, family, the media, and other environmental influences often help us create and reinforce our stereotypical perceptions and behaviors. Of course, we learn as children how to relate to the opposite sex by observing the adults in our lives, and these learned patterns often become ingrained as we grow up. The key to changing for the better is to actively identify and eliminate any negative influences that still control us.

I've developed a handy little exercise to help you accomplish this, called stereotype stimuli:

1. Read over the questions you just answered.
2. For each "yes" answer, do a little rewriting. Simply turn the question into a statement.
3. List at least two to three reasons for the belief expressed in that statement. Those reasons for your "yes" answer reflect where your thinking came from and what factors keep it going.

Here are some examples.

Question: Do you believe married men are entitled to a fling or two or three or more? Your answer: "*Yes.*"

Turn your "yes" answer into a statement: "*I believe married men are entitled to a fling or two or three or more.*"

Why do you believe this? Write the reasons down:

- *"That's what my daddy did in his marriage, so it must be okay."*
- *"That's what my daddy taught me, so it must be true."*
- *"Mom never complained, so my wife won't."*
- *"I haven't been caught; what's the big deal?"*

Question: Do you believe a man has to give up his money to get your honey? Your answer: *"Yes."*

Turn your "yes" answer into a statement: *"I believe men have to show me the money before I give up the honey."*

Why do you believe this? Write the reasons down:

- *"All brothers want is the pum-pum, so why not get paid?"*
- *"I've gotten paid pretty good."*
- *"My mama taught me I better shop around."*
- *"This is a good way to determine a man's worth."*

Question: Do you believe all men are dogs? Your answer: *"Yes."*

Turn your "yes" into a statement: *"I believe all men are dogs."*

Why do you believe this? Write your reasons down:

- *"That's what Mama and Papa told me."*
- *"My girlfriends sing that anthem; can they all be wrong?"*
- *"Look at Jesse Jackson. He's a holy man and he couldn't keep it in his pants."*

Question: Do you believe most black women are angry and difficult? Your answer: *"Yes."*

Turn your "yes" into a statement: *"I believe most black women are angry and difficult."*

Why do you believe this? Write your answers down:

- *"My mother, her mother, and all their friends were angry. Therefore, all black women must be angry."*
- *"When I go out, all I see are angry black women."*
- *"All the women I've dated are angry."*

Step 4: Flip the Script

Replace your negative behaviors or perceptions with constructive, healthy alternatives. As you learn to substitute constructive behaviors and perceptions for stereotypical, dysfunctional ones, your opportunities for productive and loving relationships automatically increase. You're now evaluating people on their actual merits, and you are behaving more authentically.

Go back to the previous exercise. Put on your thinking cap as you look over your "yes" statements and the reasons you listed for your stereotypical thoughts and actions. Here's a hugely important revelation: the reasons you listed for your stereotypical beliefs and behaviors are the beliefs that keep you stuck in this negative style of relating. If stereotypes are false, then the reasons you gave to justify them must be equally false.

Now, let's debunk each reason by "flipping the script."

Write down every possible rebuttal to each of the reasons that maintain your stereotypical thought and behavior style. These new statements will be your game plan for eliminating this aspect of our PTSD and learning new, healthier ways of interacting.

"I believe married men are entitled to a fling or two or three or more."
Reason: *That's what my daddy did in his marriage, so it must be okay.*
Rebuttal: Dad's marriage is not my marriage; I should be true to my own marriage.

Reason: *That's what my daddy taught me, so it must be true.*

Rebuttal: Just because Daddy was unfaithful doesn't make it right. Daddy was a good man, but he wasn't on it all the time.

Reason: *Mom never complained, so my wife won't.*

Rebuttal: I'm not married to Mommy. Maybe she complained but I didn't hear it. Maybe I should talk with her about the true impact of Dad's cheating.

Reason: *I haven't been caught; what's the big deal?*

Rebuttal: Just because I've gotten away with it so far doesn't mean my luck won't run out. It's better to be honest and focus my energy on my relationship.

"I believe men have to show me the money before I give up the honey."

Reason: *All the brothers want is the pum-pum, so why not get paid?*

Rebuttal: Maybe the brothers really want more. Maybe I need to bring a deeper, more substantive part of myself into my relationships.

Reason: *I've gotten paid pretty well.*

Rebuttal: Really, what did I get? A few dresses and shoes and my light bill paid once in a while. Is it worth the heartache that follows the crash and burn of yet another mercenary, superficial relationship?

Reason: *My mama taught me I better shop around.*

Rebuttal: Mama shopped around. Maybe that's why she never got married. Maybe I can do better in my relationships.

Reason: *This is a good way to determine a man's worth.*

Rebuttal: Maybe a better way to determine a man's worth is by the size of his heart, not the size of his wallet.

"I believe all men are dogs."

Reason: *That's what Mama and Papa told me.*

Rebuttal: Now that I think about it, I have known some good black men. Maybe my parents told me that out of a misguided effort to shelter me from *some* bad men.

Reason: *All my girlfriends sing that anthem; how can they all be wrong?*

Rebuttal: Maybe they are wrong. Not one of them has a really satisfying relationship. Maybe I should seek out guys who are not bowwows.

Reason: *Look at Jesse Jackson. He's a holy man and he can't keep it in his pants.*

Rebuttal: Jesse made a mistake. All people make mistakes. Jesse may be a minister, but he does not represent all brothers, and he is only human!

"I believe most black women are angry and difficult."

Reason: *My mother, my grandmother, and all their friends were angry. Therefore, all black women must be angry.*

Rebuttal: Mama is Mama. She does not represent all black women. Maybe she wasn't even as angry as I thought. Childhood memories can become warped over time. Let me speak about this with her or someone else who knew my parents.

Reason: *All I see when I go out are herds of angry sisters.*

Rebuttal: Maybe I want to perceive them as angry because their agenda does not include me. Maybe they're turned off by my tired lines. Maybe when I don't get my way with women, it's easier to dismiss them as angry. I'll give myself a reality check by actively working on my perceptions about the ladies and trying to meet them halfway.

Reason: *All the black women I've dated were angry.*

Rebuttal: Duh, maybe they were angry over my behavior. Or maybe I chose so-called angry women because of my own agenda. I'll try to flip this script by being kinder and making healthier choices.

Step 5

The final step of stereotype smashing involves daily practice. Go over your stereotype smasher exercises regularly. Read, analyze, and rewrite them as your insights deepen. Writing is a powerful thera-peutic tool. Make a daily effort to eliminate your stereotypical ways of thinking and behaving by replacing these thoughts and behaviors with the logical thinking you have generated and put in place. Do this with friends, family, loved ones, partners, potential partners, and even strangers on the street. Finally, begin behaving in ways that re-flect your new unbiased and fair minded thinking. Your new reper-toire of relationship behaviors and perceptions may feel awkward and difficult at first, but you will be soon rewarded with far more pos-itive relationship outcomes.

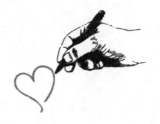

CHAPTER FIVE

THE WAR GAMES: SECRET STRATEGIES AND COUNTERINTELLIGENCE

I'll never forget a phone call I received from an irate husband during my radio show.

"Where is your loyalty?" he demanded. "Are you trying to get us in trouble? The BS you've been spreading about why we do what we do and how we're really supposed to think and act as black men is only giving the women more ammunition. If you trust them, you're out of your mind, and if you were a real brother, you wouldn't be giving up the playbook."

The husband had it dead wrong, as did other male listeners who called in to voice similar complaints. Let me assure you, I'm not giving up the playbook to ingratiate myself with the sisters, prove I'm a superior black man, or crash the ladies' male-bashing party. I'm just a firm believer in the old adage "The truth will set you free."

Most brothers can't see any reason to change their behavior and give up their secrets, because when it comes to sex and relationships in the black community, it is a man's world—at least it *appears* that way. They're wrong: our secrets and strategies are actually our greatest obstacles to greater self-understanding, true personal fulfillment, and the betterment of our community.

So, yes, I'm about to do it—reveal the black man's fondest secrets, deepest fears, desires, and self-protective strategies. The real-life case histories and examples you're about to read here are not just entertaining. They'll also help you understand why secret strategies don't really protect men or sharpen their game. The harm these secrets and strategies create goes beyond driving sisters crazy. In fact, these secrets and strategies are the black man's greatest downfall.

Now, sisters are not complete innocents either. They have their own secrets and strategies, although the black woman's game book is weighed more heavily toward defensive maneuvers—intelligence gathering and counterstrategies that sisters developed over time in order to handle the brothers. Still, not all sisters are merely defending themselves. Some women are fully capable of initiating their own offensive action, so I'll be busting out their playbook as well.

My point is that it's time for both sides in our gender war to stop dealing with the opposite sex in manipulative and self-defeating ways.

Yet not all strategies are negative. A little "game" can be healthy, like playing hard to get or waiting for a commitment before engaging in full-frontal sex.

My concern is with the strategies that keep us warring and eventually defeat us.

Secret Strategies, Intelligence Gathering, Counterstrategies, and Our PTSD

You've probably already figured out that our secrets and strategies originated as coping mechanisms to help us survive slavery and maintain our sanity. You've also jumped ahead to the realization that these defenses linger on in the form of the dysfunctional behaviors that destroy our relationships.

Many of these negative behaviors originate in what I call the "two-faced syndrome," which dates back to slavery days. One face expressed the superficial personality that the master expected. For some of us, that face represented a person who bowed, scraped, shuffled, grinned the watermelon-eating grin, and answered "yes sir" to each and every demand. This face degraded us, but it kept us out of trouble because the only way to stay safe was by hiding and protecting our true thoughts and feelings.

The second face was the one we revealed to each other as lovers, friends, and family members. The second personality was more authentic, more in alignment with our real selves, our real feelings. Yet, as the conditions of slavery eroded our relationships, that first face—that superficial, shuck-and-jive personality—began to corrupt our second, more authentic face. The manipulation and lying were no longer restricted to our interactions with the master, and our relationships with each other suffered even more damage.

Added to the negative effects of that dual personality was slavery's blow to our self-esteem. Somewhere along our journey through slavery and racism, we lost a sense of our greatness and beauty, and we've never fully recovered. A poor self-image cripples our ability to be intimate with another person, because we don't feel deserving of love and caring. We've grown so distrustful and cynical of each other's intentions that many of us believe the only way we can relate to one another without risking emotional destruction is by playing mind games—keeping secrets and employing strategies. These negative, dishonest behaviors determine the types of people we seek out and the kinds of relationships we establish with them. We believe all this espionage and game playing will protect us, but it winds up destroying our chances for happiness.

We've lost sight of what we really need and want. Instead of searching for a suitable mate with whom we can share our lives and love, we seek out fellow game players who embroil us in the kinds of relationships that dishonor both parties.

Let's take a closer look at the ways in which this romantic espionage plays out. I've divided the war games into male and female tactics. Keep in mind, though, that some strategies may be employed more frequently by men or by women, but many are the chosen weapons for both sides in our gender war.

The 411 on the Men

Fear of Black Women

One of black men's biggest secrets is that they truly fear black women's intelligence and strength. Black men are terrified by the prospect of being dominated—another legacy of PTSD—so they overcompensate by getting heavy-handed and insisting on being in charge. Yet these men secretly believe that black women—who kept the postslavery home intact when black men couldn't find work—are really in charge. Many of the black man's strategies developed to defend him from this fear of domination.

The hip-hop culture in particular raised the stakes of our male-female conflict higher than ever. Big pimpin' MCs, barely clad video girls, strippers played off as legit stage stars, and the growing urban porn industry are all manifestations of the brother's secret insecurities when it comes to love and sex. The formerly freaky is now everyday business, and love has little place in this scenario.

The current craze for knocking boots with OPP is another expression of the black man's fear of commitment and being dominated—one that enables men to hit it and quit it and still front like real men.

Randy went from office affair to office affair at the Ivy League college where he worked in the admissions department. Then he met Joan, a married professor whose husband often traveled for his own consulting business. Between the excuses of late-night research and academic meetings, Joan seemed like a great prospect for extracurricular activities.

"Why not?" Randy reasoned to himself. "She has a husband and doesn't want to leave him. She's just a little lonely and looking for some excitement. She's willing to try anything because she has nothing to lose." After four months, the passion petered out. Joan was happy to stick to her husband, and Randy moved on to Delores, an undergrad with a fiancé.

Randy had grown up with a single mom who ran through men like Bud sells beers. Randy's mom was a sexy, fun-loving woman who attracted men by the dozens, but she had little interest in settling down. So Randy witnessed countless men loving and bedding his mother, only to be "fired" as soon as she became displeased or bored. Randy began to believe that women had ultimate contol of other men and began to fear the power of his mom and women in general to easily reject these men. Though he was completely unaware of his fears, when Randy became an adult and formed his own relationships with women, he never offered genuine emotional connection. Not caring was his best defense against the certainty and fear of rejection, and Randy saw no reason why he should depart from his program of emotional detachment.

"I have everything you get from a relationship," he explained, "with none of the hassles."

Fear of Bedroom Failure

Believe it or not, the "John Shaft syndrome" can also reflect fear of failure in the bedroom: "If all I've got is penis power and it fails me, what kind of man am I?" The John Shaft bluff also protects these men from the fear of being overwhelmed by the black woman's sexuality. This is one reason why brothers have a reputation for being "selfish" in bed—"I'm finished, baby; how about you?" If he tries to please his woman and fails, he will feel inadequate, even powerless, so he spreads himself sexually among many different women. Fear of not living up to the John Shaft standard makes it nearly impossible to commit sexually to one woman who might find him lacking. If she rejected him, no other woman would be there to bolster his ego, and what kind of black stud would he be then?

Dan was the youngest of five sons, and he grew up in the shadow of his athletic older brothers. They were all big men, over six feet, with strong, husky builds, and every evening the phone constantly rang with calls from smitten young women. Short in stature, with a slim build, Dan was the odd man out in the family, and he'd seen his brothers naked enough times to know that he was not as generously endowed either.

Deep down inside, Dan believed that he could never compete with his older brothers—and, by extension, with all the other brothers out there who were more blessed by Mother Nature. How could he ever trust a sister to be faithful to him when his own family members could show her a far better time in bed?

So Dan cultivated a charming, funny personality and polished approach that would win him as many ladies as possible. No one was a bigger flirt or collected more telephone numbers than Dan, and he felt great about that. Yet Dan's relationships never worked out. His brothers had all married and become fathers, but Dan reached the age of forty and he was still out there, playing the swinging single. Dan desperately wanted a wife and children of his own, but he couldn't risk putting all his love into one woman when he just knew she would eventually become sexually bored and look for a better man. Finally, Dan took the leap and married Charise, a petite, quiet, young virgin. Their sex life seemed fine, and Charise blessed Dan with twin boys, but Dan couldn't trust her love. He had never stopped flirting madly with every attractive female he met, but as his insecurities deepened, he took it further. He bedded the secretary of an associate and began picking women up at clubs on Friday nights. It wasn't long before Charise did leave Dan for another man—not because this new man had larger sexual equipment but because he had the ability to love her and be faithful.

Mama's Boy

Another secret zealously guarded by black men is that they measure the worth of every woman they meet according to the standard of care they *believe* they received from their mothers. Because of the widespread absence of the black father in our homes—yet another aspect of our PTSD—many black men never make the necessary emotional break from their mothers that will enable them to transfer their identification to their father. This is supposed to happen at an appropriate developmental stage, around twelve or thirteen years old. When there's no father figure present, the transfer can't take place, and the boy doesn't separate from his mother. No matter who she really was or how she really behaved, Mama remains that first love, an ideal figure in her son's mind: "Don't you talk about my mama!" No real-life woman ever measures up to Mama, and that maternal tie can keep him from committing to a real-life woman. No woman is good enough, compared to Mama!

My Woman Lets Me Do It

Another secret black men don't want their women to discover is that most black men cheat because their women allow it! Infidelity is the most common issue that brings couples to my office. In some cases the woman is unfaithful, but most of the time the man is the cheater. Some unfaithful men show absolute callousness toward their partners' feelings. They'll stay out all night and allow outside women to call their home telephone. You could say these brothers are very sloppy, yet most of them are pretty sophisticated, although not as slick as their women, as you will soon discover when you read some of their stories. One reason for these men's sloppiness is that they have to juggle too many details, so some evidence gets away from them. But the main reason they leave a trail of glaring evidence is because their women give them tacit permission to play outside the yard.

Most women don't say anything, but it's understood that "What I don't know won't hurt me." Nona actually encouraged her husband to have sex when she was six months pregnant with their second child. Four years earlier, when Nona was undergoing the difficult pregnancy that resulted in their son, her husband became so frustrated that he started drinking. The drinking led to womanizing that continued for the first few months of their son's life, while Nona was still recuperating from childbirth. Nona had been forbidden to have sex for the remainder of her second pregnancy, and she feared Balford would repeat his reckless behavior, putting herself and her children at risk for HIV and other diseases.

Desperate, Nona asked her sister Mae, who was also married, albeit a bad marriage, to sleep with Balford. At first, her sister was horrified by the request. Not only would she be violating her own marriage vows, but she'd also be sexing her own sister's husband. But Nona begged, and finally, Mae reluctantly agreed.

Balford was also taken aback by his wife's suggestion. Nona insisted, though, and they all finally decided that Mae would visit Balford at his and Nona's home on Mae's husband's bowling night.

That evening, Nona went to the movies and tried to concentrate on the Eddie Murphy movie on the screen. When she returned, Balford was parked in front of the television set, silent and sullen. They'd decided beforehand that they wouldn't mention what had gone on while Nona was out and her sister was there. But Balford finally burst out that he felt humiliated and pimped. "If I need sex that badly, I'll go to a ho'," he said. "That's just what I don't want you to do, darling; can't you see?" Nona told him.

She asked Mae to continue taking care of her husband's needs, but Mae was hesitant to discuss it. Yet they were obviously getting it on, and liking it more. Over the next few months, whenever Nona left the home so Mae could service her husband, she began finding more and more evidence that duty had become a pleasure: an empty champagne bottle in the recycling bin, heavily perfumed sheets crushed in the hamper, a bouquet of flowers under the coffee grounds in the garbage, a crumpled bill in the wastebasket from the expensive restaurant Nona and her husband frequented on special occasions only. Meanwhile, Balford grew more and more distant. Nona delivered another son, and two months later, Mae and Balford ran off together. They left a note in which they told Nona that they were sorry to hurt her, but she had to bear her share of the responsibility for what happened. Thanks to Nona, they had fallen in love.

Brothers' Secret Strategies

My Friday evening group for men is a microcosm of the brothers' world, and we deal with cheating more than any other issue. I've accumulated enough information to present you with an FBI manual on the strategies brothers employ to get over on females. The strategies and stories you're about to read are real; the names have been changed to protect the guilty and innocent alike.

The Mission: Cheating Without Being Caught

Brothers in committed relationships put a lot of time and effort into scoring as many women as possible or maintaining a main outside squeeze on the side without being caught. Some of these strategies can be pretty bizarre.

Strategies: hanging with the homeboyz

A favorite tactic is calling on the brotherhood to cover our tracks. We tell our girl or wife that we're at a buddy's house watching the fight when we're really out with the boys chasing other women or fighting a new conquest over her drawers.

No one had more running buddies or a supposedly busier sports schedule than Devin. Saturdays were devoted to hoops, then discussing the game with the other players at the sports bar. Sundays were spent watching pro games at various friends' houses. At night, Devin took in the action at the horse races or played cards. Then there were those weekend trips to Vegas or wherever else a major fight was taking place.

Devin was a sports aficionado, a walking compendium of facts on legendary contests in all sports and on the biographical and performance data of his favorite athletes. Devin also genuinely enjoyed the company of his friends. His wife was used to his obsession with sports and never questioned her husband's whereabouts. But Devin was a liar. His busy schedules and sports activities were all fake! His real sport took place between the sheets with women who were not his wife, and his elaborate schedule of activities and wide network of male buddies were often a ruse to help him keep up his secret game.

The cell phone

The cell phone is the cheating black man's electronic enabler of covert communications with outside females. (Of course, single females who want to avoid adulterous brothers should know that when he gives you his cell phone number only, he's up to no good.) These men avoid trouble at home by switching their cell phone to "silent" or "vibrate," so the wife or main partner has no idea when he gets calls. Those brothers often glue themselves to their cell phones to maintain contact with the outside women, telling their suspicious wives that "it's business."

Lester had the dopest cell phone out there—Internet access, electronic casino, video games, and enough memory to store sixty-plus phone numbers of the outside women he'd bedded over the past three years. Each woman was assigned her own code, he explained. This system enabled Lester to identify each caller and decide whether to answer the phone or, if his wife or another female was nearby, to leave it alone. Lester not only cheated on his wife; he also played around on his girlfriends. Lester liked to joke that his wife always complained that he spent weeknights and weekends on the front porch, talking incessantly into his cell phone. "Who the hell are you talking to?" she'd always ask. "My boys," he'd answer. "Can't you let a brother bond with his buddies?"

The business trip

This is the opportunity a cheating brother lives for. The strategy is to inform the spouse or partner with deep regret that the boss says he has to take this trip alone. Now the way is clear to meet new women and stay out all night without having to concoct an excuse. Or he can bring along a girlfriend for a few days of penalty-free sex and fun on the town without fearing that someone who knows his wife will spot them. A smart brother never books the girl's flight on his credit card: either she pays for it and he reimburses her, or he simply pays cash for her ticket.

Reggie volunteered for every business trip that came up on the job. He liked to recount for the group his adventures in one particular town he visited several times a year. Reggie was especially tickled that he'd acquired a "second, unofficial wife" in that city, because he didn't have to shell out the expense of bringing a girl with him. His "second wife" missed him so much that he was guaranteed hot sex and deluxe treatment whenever he visited. And his real wife was so jumpy over the possibility that he might be tempted to cheat on these trips that she treated him like the King of Siam. "Wife number two" knew about wife number one, but wife number one hadn't a clue about her competition.

The wedding band protocols

This one is not so secret, but most members of the cheating brotherhood follow this protocol when they're on the prowl: If you want to move freely, remove the wedding band. The really bold brother employs reverse psychology. He purposely wears a wedding band, even if he's not married, because that little bit of gold lends the extra added attraction of not appearing to be on the prowl. Some women lower their defenses, providing more opportunity for him to get over, while the flash of gold lures those women who welcome the challenge of hard-to-get men. Other brothers flaunt a wedding band as a way to declare that any woman who deals with them can expect nothing but sex.

Joshua's flaunting of his platinum wedding band matched the cool, laid-back attitude that so many ladies seemed to find irresistible. All he had to do was flash his winning grin, framed by matching dimples, at a likely prospect, and he was in. Joshua enjoyed the game of magnetizing a female so that she was drawn to move next to him at a bar. He'd chat her up in a friendly but non-committal tone, even casually mentioning his wife and children, then gaze deep into her eyes for a moment before looking off at another woman. He liked to confuse her: reel her in, let the line back out, then bring her back in again, until she was hooked. He explained to his boys that women were drawn to his contradictory behavior. It disarmed them, plus—and this was the real ploy, he always noted—women react strongly to the threat of competition. Those casual glances at other females made the woman by his side even more determined that no other woman in the place would get him.

Working late and business dinners

We all know a brother has to work hard to make a living. The beauty is that working overtime is a perfect excuse for spending time outside the home with other females. The efficient brother creates a schedule that weaves in his professional, family, and extracurricular-love lives so that he gets maximum quality experiences within the briefest amount of time possible.

Sebastian was an attorney who kept late hours, but "working late" often meant he was taking off briefs, not preparing them. I don't believe I've ever encountered another man who worked as much or played as hard. I'll never forget the time he outlined his typical weekday cheating schedule for our men's group:

Monday:	9 A.M. to noon	court
	Noon to 1 P.M.	lunch—Ingrid
	1:30 P.M. to 5 P.M.	office
	5 P.M. to 7 P.M.	cocktails—Melba
	7 P.M. to 9 P.M.	dinner—Trish
	9 P.M. to 10:30 P.M.	motel—Ingrid ("first hired, last retired")
	10:30 P.M.	home—lie to wife about day's events

Sebastian thrived on the adrenaline of his hectic double life, and he pulled off his tricky schedule with no other aids but a reliable Rolex, a palm pilot, daily herbs and vitamins, and a great sense of timing.

Just friends

If friendship is a normal part of human existence, why should a brother abandon his female friends or stop making new ones just because he's married or committed? At least, that's the argument the guys in the men's group have presented. "Just friends" is part strategy, part denial, and all hard-to-defeat alibi. It's also the most commonly used lie to mask cheating. If the man is spotted or even busted with the other woman, he simply says she's just a friend.

In a variation on this strategy, the brother says he's going out with a "friend" but neglects to mention the friend is female. Brothers have relied on this strategy for so long that they've managed to convince themselves that these friendships are completely innocent, even though they often escalate into infidelities. They even persuade themselves that "this time, I'll be a good boy," every time they make a new "friend." Of course, that promise lasts as long as the first peek at her cleavage, the first brushing together of hands, or the first deep look into her eyes.

Stanley was the master flirt of the group, a man with many, many female friends and a class act for his wife. Stanley never referred to these women as conquests; they were always his friends! Whenever his wife questioned these friendships, Stanley made her feel guilty about her suspicions. How could she accuse him of cheating when she knew what a friendly fellow he was, a writer who was naturally curious about people, including women? Did she want to cut him off from other human beings, the stuff of his work and his life? In fact, Stanley even convinced himself that he was just a very friendly man—nothing more. Yet these friendships invariably heated up into affairs.

During the time Stanley was meeting with the men's group, he formed a new friendship with a fellow writer named Vanessa, a new member of his fiction workshop. Vanessa was particularly supportive of Stanley's work and always offered accolades when he read the latest installment on his second novel for the group. For his part, Stanley was happy to mentor the less experienced Vanessa and meet her for extra help outside the workshop. After a few weeks, Vanessa suggested that it would be more convenient for both of them if they met in her studio apartment. She didn't want Stanley to keep shelling out for their coffee and pastries. After all, hosting him was the least she could do in exchange for his help.

Stanley came to the men's group one night looking shamefaced. He confessed: that week, during their third writing session, he had wound up in bed with Vanessa. He just couldn't understand how things had gotten so out of control. All he wanted to do was help a younger writer, but Vanessa had developed a crush on her idol and he just couldn't resist all that adoration. The other members of the therapy group didn't buy Stanley's story. To a man, they all pointed out that the initial friendship was really Stanley's MO for working his way up to sex. If he was insisting his relationships were innocent, he was also fooling himself.

It wasn't me

The perpetrator of this strategy knows exactly what he's doing. He just denies it to his wife or steady girlfriend. No matter what kind of situation this brother is caught in, he denies what his wife's own eyes are telling her. Some brothers are so skilled at this ploy that their wives or partners begin to doubt what they've seen: "Maybe I was so upset that it just *looked* like they were naked in bed together."

Harry's wife almost caught him out on at least a dozen occasions, and each time he convinced her "it wasn't me." Finally, he was caught butt naked with his lover. Can you believe he used the "it wasn't me" defense and it worked?

Here's what happened. Harry had promised to take Cara, his wife, out on the town for her birthday, but instead he sent flowers to her office with a note that read, "Happy birthday, honey. I have to meet a client tonight. So sorry. I'll make it up to you—promise. Don't wait up."

Cara telephoned her best friend to cry on her shoulder, and they decided to celebrate the occasion with a nice dinner and kicking it at a local club. They had a great time, and as they left and were pulling away from the curb, they noticed Harry's car parked in front of a nearby house. Cara and her friend swung into action. They marched up to the house and banged on the door, screaming, "Fire! Fire!" A barely clad and terrified woman opened the door. They burst past her, hunting for the bedroom, where they found Cara's husband naked on the woman's bed.

Harry was belly laughing as he told the men's group that he persuaded his wife that he'd taken too much of an antidepressant medication and was in some sort of fugue state. This strange woman had been sitting at a nearby restaurant as he was having dinner with his client. She'd obviously fixated on him. He took his pill after dinner, and, in his confusion, he allowed this stranger to take him home and remove his clothes. He was not guilty, by reason of drug-induced temporary insanity: "It wasn't *the real* me!" Cara bought this bold defense that earned him the nickname in the group of "Harry Houdini."

I only did it once

This is a more common strategy that's often used the first time brothers are caught red-handed. These brothers admit to their guilt, because they know their penalty will be probation rather than exile. In fact, smart brothers who really want to protect their relationship will cut their losses once they're caught out and retire from the cheating game. Most plead their case by insisting this was the first and only time they cheated, but they've usually been cheating for some time. Why turn over evidence of prior indiscretions if she's got no proof?

It won't happen again

Ironically, this strategy is a favorite of habitual offenders who promise never to cheat again but keep on doing exactly what they've been doing. They just refine their game to make it slicker, while at the same time they have the chutzpa to promise they'll do better and it won't ever happen again.

When Diane presented her live-in boyfriend Earl with solid evidence of his affair with Lea, he begged and pleaded for forgiveness as fat, salty tears rolled down his face. Lea meant nothing to him; he didn't even know why he'd allowed himself to be tempted. Diane was everything to him. He couldn't live without her, if only she'd give him another chance.

Earl seemed to be behaving himself for the next several months—at least, Diane had no proof to the contrary. Then, two weeks before they were due to fly to Cincinnati to visit her parents, Diane received a phone call from a woman named Beverly, who claimed to be having an affair with Earl. Beverly wanted Earl, she informed Diane in no uncertain terms, and she meant to move him from Diane's apartment to her own. When Beverly dropped a few choice bits of information regarding Earl's anatomy, Diane knew she wasn't lying.

She confronted Earl when he got home from work that night, and he immediately caved in and admitted that he'd gotten drunk one night and wound up sleeping with Beverly. In fact, he didn't even remember her name until Diane mentioned it. Beverly must have picked through his pockets and found their home number, he theorized. She was nothing to him, and he was so very sorry. Diane was adamant; she wanted Earl out. But he suddenly ran out their door and onto their apartment building's roof. As Diane watched in horror, Earl stood near the edge, threatening to jump if she didn't forgive him and take him back. He swore on his own mother's life that he would never stray again. Life was for learning, and he'd learned his lesson for good. Wowed by this emotional display of his love, Diane forgave Earl once again and took him back.

Sisters' Counterstrategies Against Men Who Cheat

I deliberately saved the endings to the stories you just read about brothers behaving badly and apparently getting away with it because I want to emphasize that sooner or later, every one of these brothers was busted. A man's secret strategy is rarely a match for a woman's intelligence gathering and counterstrategies. In each of the above cases, it was just a matter of time before their ladies discovered what was up and moved their men to the doghouse or kicked them to the curb. Unbeknownst to each man, the woman's counterintelligence involved gathering information slowly and painstakingly, until an airtight case was prepared and she could prosecute and lay down the law. No one matches the espionage and prosecutorial skills of a sister who believes she's being played.

Detective work

Paperwork, interviewing, surveillance, and female intuition are the sisters' strong suits. A woman will remove, Xerox, and then file the love notes and suspicious business cards she finds in her husband's briefcase, wallet, or pocket. Then, she'll replace the evidence so he never knows what happened. The woman knows just what questions to ask the credit card company. Her friend in the phone company helps identify the woman whose number keeps cropping up on the cell phone bill. The wife will visit the woman and tell her everything. Or, if she enjoys her work, the wife will call the woman with a message to meet her husband at such-and-such corner. Of course, the wife shows up instead and gets as much information as she can before revealing, "He's married—to me!" The wife will send a friend you don't know on a surveillance mission to discover if you really wound up where you said you'd be. Women will dig and dig, like a dog trying to unearth a treasured bone, until they come up with the evidence.

Several men in the group related chilling tales of being hit with all the documented evidence: reams of phone records, love notes, credit card bills—even photographs. All were amazed and shocked by the sophisticated level of their women's counterintelligence. Many of the surveillance tactics were not only bold and inspired but also brave.

Willem claimed that he just couldn't help it. Women's mouths watered whenever he was near. He was dangerously handsome, and he enjoyed all the female attention. In the ten years he'd been married, he'd had much more than his secretary, but he'd always gotten away with it. He made up for his philandering with extra-special gifts to his wife: a sapphire ring, a gold bracelet, a diamond necklace. His wife had grown up in a large family, where there was little money to make a fuss over each child's birthday or Christmas. Her weakness was those special occasions, and Willem scored big points for making a big deal over her birthday or their anniversary. Willem was proud of his wife's devotion, though that didn't keep him from bedding as many women as possible.

He was even proud when he related how his wife finally caught him cheating. She sat in a rented car outside his girlfriend's house for three consecutive nights, waiting for him to pay a visit. On the third night, he arrived. His wife took a ladder out of the car trunk and climbed up to the girl's bedroom window to take Polaroid photographs of them together. Once the images were clear, the wife rang the doorbell and confronted them with evidence, not just of this affair, but with other proof she'd already accumulated that Willem was engaged in other relationships at the same time. Willem lost the girlfriend, the other girls, and his long-suffering wife.

Forensic evidence

Women are expert forensic examiners, able to spot the tiniest telltale sign of cheating on a man's clothes and body. If this is the only proof she can get, she'll take it to trial and swiftly pass sentence.

Just about every man in my group has related how his woman hunts for evidence on clothes, in briefcases, and on the body. One girlfriend was an expert at finding hairs that weren't her own. Another had a keen sense of smell that allowed her to detect alien perfume or the lingering scent of sex. One wife could locate suspicious stains on her man's clothing.

Sandra was particularly sensitive to odors, and she was crazy about her man Julio's scent. She couldn't get enough of him, especially when he smelled of the clean, manly sweat produced by their lovemaking. Sandra suspected that Julio was getting it on with a coworker at the large corporation in San Diego where he was an account executive and she was a secretary, but he staunchly dismissed her accusations as ridiculous.

Sandra was presented with the opportunity to act as her own sleuth when she drew the coworker's name as secret Santa for the company's annual Christmas barbecue. Sandra went to the Body Shop and asked the salesperson for their most obscure perfume. The girl was delighted with her gift, and Sandra sat back and waited for the evidence to present itself.

Almost two weeks later, Julio came home late from a department seminar. Sandra wrapped him up in a long, tight squeeze and surreptitiously sniffed a few key places. Not only did she detect that fresh-hay scent of his sweat, but his body also bore the lingering trace of his coworker's new perfume. That was evidence enough to convince Sandra her man was cheating. She packed her bags and left that night.

The Mission: A One-Night Stand or First-Time Sex

Whether committed, married, or single, the majority of brothers work a battery of strategies to get a woman into bed. He'll tell her it's not about sex. It's about a way to express his genuine feelings, even his love. He'll run his motor mouth until he convinces her that giving up her sex is the right thing to do. He may make a reluctant woman his special project and devote all the time, effort, and attention it takes to conquer her. He will beg, borrow, and steal for it. He will exaggerate and tell every lie imaginable; he'll even pledge his undying love and devotion. He will work to destabilize her mind so she trusts him more than she trusts herself. He promises to deliver the world and even stick around afterward. But it's not even about bedding her. It's about winning, making that conquest, proving he's a man. Once he gets what he wanted, he loses interest and goes off to conquer new territories. Sisters need to keep in mind that all men suffer from this defect to some degree, so if a woman gives it up too quickly, she risks the chance that the man will shop but not stop.

Here are some tired lines brothers are still using to score:

I think I love you.
Of course I'll respect you in the morning.
I'll call you tomorrow.

I'll see you tomorrow.

This is the end of a beautiful friendship and the beginning of a great love affair.

You're the most gorgeous woman I ever saw.

Sex will bring us closer; it'll be good for the relationship.

If we don't do it, I'm going to explode.

If you really cared, you'd make love with me.

Sisters' Counterstrategies Against One-Night Stands and First-Time Sex

Let's get real: If a sister really likes a guy, she wants sex just as badly. The difference is that she may be more willing to wait until they get to know each other or until there's commitment. Some women are even willing to wait until marriage. Women tend to have more self-control, so their counterstrategy is all about mustering enough willpower to keep the libido in check and fend off the brother until the time is right.

Here are some favorite verbal tactics:

You can go only so far

She gives in to her passion . . . a little. She contents herself with measured doses of sexual activity, but the brother wants it all now, now, now! There may be a lot of foreplay, but matters won't go further. She may be frustrated by the waiting game, but not nearly as much as the brother. She wants to know whether the man wants her body or her love. *You can go only so far* is not so much a manipulation but a healthy, self-preserving strategy that can lead to a genuine, long-term relationship. In fact, I think it's a great idea to wait until you really know someone before you jump into bed.

Kylie Elisabeth was crazy about the very persistent Leonard, but she couldn't be sure of his intentions. He was everything she wanted in a serious partner, the perfect mate—intelligent, handsome, and hardworking; and he didn't seem to care about those forty extra pounds she carried. When they went out to dinner, he encouraged her to eat as much as she wanted, and he liked to present her with little gifts: a book she'd mentioned, a box of chocolates, flowers sent to her job. Leonard seemed like the most romantic man in the world, and he wanted to "take" her now! Kylie Elisabeth told Leonard that she wanted to wait before making love, because she'd been hurt in the past by men who had declared honorable intentions but wound up playing her.

In fact, Kylie Elisabeth was holding back at my suggestion. She had allowed herself to be used in the past, and she needed to create a more solid relationship before she became intimate again. It was difficult to deny her own desire, but Kylie Elisabeth managed to hold out for a month, during which she saw Leonard every night. By the time they finally made love, they'd established a bond based on compatibility and respect, and their lovemaking was far more passionate and tender than it would have been if they'd gotten busy the very first night they dated. Sex became a way of deepening the relationship they already enjoyed, and after a year, they married.

I'll give you what you want if you give me what I want

What she wants could be time, attention, love, or material objects. This sophisticated countermove can be powerful psychological warfare, and, unlike *you can go only so far*, this strategy does not help create stronger, more authentic relationships. The brother believes the bargain will hold: If he gives her whatever she wants, he will get what he wants. But sisters who play it this way don't always keep to the bargain.

The harder Brian tried to woo Patricia and the more he gave her, the further away she dangled that carrot. Brian whined, begged, cajoled, and nagged, until Patricia finally decided that no gift and no amount of money was worth having to put up with Brian. Brian admitted to the group that this scenario had played out in his life several times before. He had no idea what he was doing wrong. The women seemed interested in him at first, and Brian was no fool. He knew that a good part of his appeal was due to his fat wallet. He didn't mind: as long as he could pay for their attentions, it was okay with him. But Brian was crude and obvious in his tactics. The group was finally able to help him understand that his constant begging and pressuring for sex only revealed his true motives. Smart women saw through him. They knew he just wanted sex, so they paid him back by extracting as much money and as many presents as they could. Brian came across as a needy, spoiled crybaby, and sisters who never intended to give it up worked him for dinner, clothes, and cash. One particularly skilled schemer worked him so expertly well, making bedroom promises she never intended to fulfill, that she got a brand-new car.

The Mission: Living off a Sister

Some brothers have no qualms whatsoever about manipulating women for a free ride. Some of these craven men even consider this informal pimping to be their full-time job. This pimp loves to brag that he's never relied on the sweat of his own brow. All his basic needs—and essential luxuries—are funded by hardworking women. Like any other all-American pimp, these brothers prey on vulnerable women with poor self-esteem and a history of failed relationships. The brother uses serious psychology to bring a woman down even lower until she believes her sole purpose in life is to take care of her man. It doesn't go so far as real pimping—putting a woman on the street to sell her body—but the outcome is nearly as bad. These brothers rob women not only of money but also of self-respect.

Strategies: positive reinforcement

A favorite trick is positive reinforcement: every time the woman pulls out her checkbook or wallet, she gets her man's sweet words or loving. The implication is that she may have failed in other aspects of her life, but when it comes to how to treat her man, she's a resounding success. This pimp also persuades her that no one else understands or cares for her, and he does his best to keep her away from friends or family members who see through his game. All brothers who play women have a little pimp in them, but these full-out pimps may be the worst of all. They lack any spark of kindness or compassion.

Rudy's main woman, Alana, was abandoned by alcoholic parents at the age of seven and raised by a penny-pinching grandmother. Alana often lacked money for schoolbooks, wore hand-me-down clothes, and was told to put cardboard in her shoes when the soles wore out. She'd have to walk half a mile to wait for the school bus in those flimsy shoes in the freezing cold and snow of Buffalo, New York. When her grandmother died alone in her poorly heated, drafty shack of a house, Alana found plastic baggies of cash secreted behind the peeling wallpaper, in gaping wall panels, and in other secret locations. Her grandmother had squirreled away nearly fifty thousand dollars by scrimping and doing without, and by forcing her granddaughter to do the same.

Now that Alana had a comfortable bank account, in addition to her hefty salary as a registered nurse, she was able to support her man, Rudy, in the style to which he and his kind always aspire. Every time Alana handed over cash or bought him a significant gift, Rudy reinforced her generosity by looking tenderly into her eyes and telling her how proud he was of her, and what a remarkable achievement it was to overcome the legacy of stinginess in her family and be so generous. Hearing that she was so different from her grandmother was reward enough for Alana.

Put the house in both our names

This is such a common strategy, I'm surprised sisters still fall for it. Of course, this tactic comes with an arsenal of other strategies that set up naive females for the kill. The object is to weaken the woman's reason with psychological warfare so the brother can then talk her into putting the house, car, or other property in both their names, even if her money paid for it. He convinces her to open a joint account and give him signatory power. Why would she do these things? The pimp claims he loves her more than anyone else does, and the best way she can return his love is by sharing with an open heart! If you want to observe this strategy being executed by masters, head down to the beaches of Jamaica and watch the "rent-a-dreads" at work.

One rent-a-dread from Negril named Lytton convinced his woman from Chicago that he wouldn't be able to get a visitor's visa to the United States unless he could prove to the immigration authorities that he had a sizeable bank account, land, and a house. Tina, who earned a lot of money off the books from her job as an exotic dancer, was only too happy to comply. She didn't want any other tourists flying down to Jamaica to caress her man's rippling, cocoa brown muscles or running their fingers through his dreadlocks. When she went back home to work and get the money together, she was introduced to another woman who'd just spent a year teaching yoga in the same Jamaican village. The yoga teacher knew Lytton and had watched him operate with various female tourists over the course of a year. She warned Tina that he was a scam artist like other men in that village, and she shouldn't throw her money away. Lisa didn't want to hear it. She just figured the yoga teacher was jealous and couldn't understand the love Lisa shared with her island man. She went ahead with her plans to transfer her savings account from an American bank to a new account Lytton opened in his own name at a British-owned bank with branches in Jamaica. Not long after, Lytton inherited two acres of land in an up-and-coming tourist area, and Tina was only too happy to spend fifteen thousand dollars to put up small cabins equipped with showers and toilets so Lytton could prove that he had a working business in Jamaica.

One day, she was down in Jamaica visiting Lytton before his papers had come through to enter the United States, when a strange white woman drove up to their property in a new Toyota. Strapped into the back was a light-skinned boy of about six months who bore an obvious resemblance to Lytton. Gertie, Lytton's woman from Germany, had decided to pay her man a surprise visit, bearing his surprise gifts: his son and the new Toyota.

I'll do my part as soon as I get it together

This strategy involves telling the woman who's providing the brother with food, shelter, clothing, and whatever else he needs that as soon as his friend repays the loan, or that court case is won, or the backers come through for his surefire project, he'll take care of business. In fact, if she'd just invest a little more in his wardrobe, he could find a position worthy of his talents. Whenever his ship comes in, she won't have to pay for a thing. He'll take care of her in style. Of course, the ship never pulls into the harbor. These manipulators never do right.

Millie married Alvin as soon as she turned sixteen, as a way to escape the horrors of her life with a drunken, abusive father and a terrified, helpless mother. She studied for her GED and then graduated with an associates degree from her local community college. Alvin worked some nights at the local Mickey D's and tried to go to mechanics school in the morning, but he had trouble getting up early enough to be there on time, and he soon dropped out. He didn't want to be a mechanic anyway; plus, that night job was killing him, Alvin told Millie. He saw himself more as a computer salesman, but he needed to be a full-time student in order to focus on his studies. Millie saved enough money for tuition from her job as an assistant librarian, and Alvin enrolled in a computer studies program. He lasted two months, then complained that the teachers were incompetent and "didn't like me."

Several months went by, with Alvin getting more and more tied up with the boys of the ghetto. He was thinking about his future, Alvin told Millie. He didn't want to make any more rash mistakes. When he finally found the right work, she could quit her job and they'd live in style. He never did find the right work.

Don't pressure me!

Some users go on the attack if their women apply pressure. "Of course I'm trying to get a job; stop nagging!" Actually, finding a job *is* his job, and that requires energy and focus, so back off and give a brother his respect! By the way, if this brother actually does land a job, you can be sure he won't accept it, or he'll work for a brief period before he quits because the work is beneath him! In Alvin's case, the next career move was fame as a hip-hop star, and he began spending less time looking for work and more time busting rhymes in his friend's basement "studio."

As the months dragged on into a year, Millie began to challenge Alvin. He needed to grow up and make up his mind to study something—anything! It wasn't fair that she was supporting both of them on her meager salary. With each demand to mobilize, Alvin became more and more sullen and withdrawn. Soon, Millie was afraid to say anything to him. At the first tentative question about what he'd done that day, Alvin would jump up from the couch and disappear into his friend's "studio" for the entire night. Finally, he left one day while she was at work, clearing out her TV and stereo system. He'd found another woman who wasn't wise to his game.

I'm struggling to find myself

This spin-off of the *don't pressure me* strategy elevates the brother's quest for a simple job into a struggle to find his true place in this cruel and crazy world. Once this manipulator figures out his destiny, the right career will come, and his woman will luxuriate in a lifestyle she's never even imagined possible.

Alvin played off his laziness as a search for himself. Becoming a mechanic or working in computers were forms of prostitution for a man as gifted as Alvin. Why couldn't Millie ease up and support his dream? Didn't she realize that when he made it, she would live like a queen?

Everybody's against a brother

How can a brother land a job that isn't degrading in this racist world? There's a conspiracy against black men, and if a woman nags a brother to find work, she is insensitive to his pain and not supporting "The Cause." If she were a true black sister, she would understand what he's up against. Nothing is more insulting to a black woman than being labeled a race traitor. In reality, the man is taking out his PTSD anger on the woman and using racism as an excuse for his personal failures.

Tyrone was a fifty-something-year-old sometime truck driver with a wife and children who were fed up with decades of enduring his rants about The Man, and how The Man keeps a brother down. Over the course of their entire marriage, Marta, Tyrone's wife, had put up with this excuse for his erratic work habits, his accusations that she wasn't supportive of her black husband, and his lingering foul moods. Now that her three children were nearly grown, she saw no reason to spend her golden years tied to this albatross. In fact, when her last child graduated high school and moved out to room with other friends attending a nearby college, Marta packed up all Tyrone's worldly belongings and moved him in her own car to his older sister's home two hours away.

Marta had stuck with Tyrone all those years because she didn't want her children to suffer as she had from the absence of a father. She expected their children to be heartbroken, even though they were old enough to take care of themselves, but, to her surprise, they were almost as relieved about the separation as she was. In fact, each child told Marta that they wished she'd done it much earlier, that living with all that tension had to have been worse than having a part-time dad.

Look what I'm giving you

Some brothers actually believe that their sex is worth the cost of keeping them in style. This man will actually tell a sister that his stuff is so good—and so many other females are begging for it!—it's worth the price.

Roy was my male therapy group's ranking ladies' man. He claimed he never had to work, unless he needed to rustle up extra cash to woo a new lady. Roy loved to brag that women bought all his clothing, and one married woman even gifted him with a flashy sports car. Roy attributed his great success as a gigolo to skillful employment of all the strategies we covered, plus convincing all his women that contributing to his welfare was the very least they could do, because the reward of his great sex was priceless. Roy often boasted to the other men that these women always said he was the best they ever had, and he had no qualms about preening to these women about the great gift he was giving them. Believe it or not, women fell for that line, and the constant threat of competition led each one to do all she could to make sure she wouldn't have to share his gift.

I have to admit that most of us were jealous of Roy's mackin'. Later on, though, we discovered there was more to his story than Roy was telling. I'm about to share that information in the next section, the sisters' counterstrategies.

The Sisters' Counterstrategies Against Men Who Live off Women

Usually, a sister doesn't mind shelling out a little money, especially if she believes she's getting equal value in return. But when a woman suspects her man is a liar and manipulator or has another sugar mama, she initiates any of the following defenses:

Cancel the credit cards.
Stop paying on the car.
Take him to court for his half of the mortgage.
Throw his clothes out the window or even shred or burn them.
Show up at his job, if he has one, and out him.

Roy, the ladies' man, was busted out when his fiancée asked her best friend to do a stakeout across the street from Roy's apartment building on a Friday night he was supposed to leave for a weekend with his mom in Omaha. When Roy stepped out the front door, he wasn't carrying a suitcase. The friend followed Roy as he drove to a house two miles away. He rang the bell, and a woman answered the door. The next night, Roy paid a visit to a different woman's home. Roy's girlfriend now had proof that she was part of an all-female relief effort—RWF, or Roy's Welfare Fund. Not only did the fiancée cut off Roy without warning, she also let the two outside women know what was up. The fiancée even had enough money left in the bank to pay a thug to administer a licking Roy would not soon forget. Fortunately, Roy recovered with no lasting damage, except to his ego.

The 411 on the Women

Women Play Just As Well As Men, If not Better!

As I stated earlier, most of the black woman's intelligence gathering goes toward formulating defensive behaviors—counterstrategies to defeat the men's missions. Yet women also initiate disturbing and destructive strategies.

A cheating woman could teach a faithless man a trick or two. All women, black women included, are far better than any man at covering their tracks and presenting a game face. Women are socialized to be meek, quiet, dependent followers. This helps them evolve ways to get what they want or need by covert, indirect means. Through necessity, women have learned to outplay the original players.

A woman's biggest secret could even be that she welcomes the challenge of a difficult man in order to prove that she's the better player. She may cry to her auntie, cousin, mama, and all her friends about how much she longs for a sensitive, understanding, and caring brother. But when that kind, mild brother shows up at her doorstep, nine times out of ten she is soon bored and ready to trade him in for the challenge of a bad boy. She wants to be the sole female—the best hunter in the pack—to tame this wild one.

Pam bored the tears out of the women in her carpool every morning as they drove together to work. She was always regaling them with sob stories about her long, sleepless nights of touring the city's bars, looking for her errant boyfriend, Donald. Or about how he flirted with some actress in the play he was rehearsing. Or how he gave her money whenever he felt like it, which wasn't often enough. Yet whenever someone dared to suggest that Pam cut her losses and run, she reacted defensively. How could she leave him? They were in love; the man was just going through a phase. He'd soon straighten out. In fact, Donald eventually left Pam for another woman, the actress in his new play. No more bad boys, Pam vowed. She was going for a man of substance, one with a kind heart and a good character.

Roma, one of her girlfriends, had just the man for Pam—her cousin Valentine, who had recently moved to town from Atlanta. Valentine was a great catch, a widower who had tragically lost his young wife in a car crash three years earlier. Valentine was kind, funny, attractive, and ambitious. He had just opened his own garage at a busy intersection and was sure to do a booming business.

Pam tried with Valentine. He was sweet and attentive, but she found herself bored and empty. Where was the challenge? Pam was kidding only herself when she cried to anyone who would listen that all she wanted was a good man. Women often accuse men of being hunters who quit the game after they've nabbed their prey, but Pam was a huntress herself, out to prove that she was the woman who could come away with the big game.

LOVE PRESCRIPTION

What's Love Got to Do with It?

Here's another secret that women don't want men to know: Despite the insistence by men that the double standard is a fact of nature, that only males are capable of hitting it and quitting it, women are perfectly capable of sex without commitment.

It had been eight months since Kamara broke off with Ben, and her sex life was nonexistent. When Jerome, the young plumber sent by the landlord to fix her bathtub faucet, began calling almost every night after the eleven o'clock news to ask if they could hang out, she finally said okay.

Much to her surprise, that was all Kamara and Jerome did—make small talk, watch a late movie, and drink a few beers. When he called again and asked to see her, Kamara complained to a friend. "What's he about?" she wanted to know. "Maybe he wants to get to know you first," her friend suggested. "I already know myself," Kamara snapped back. "I want a man in my bed, that's my RESPECT!" The next time Jerome called, Kamara asked why he'd refused her bed. He shyly said something about wanting to take his time so they wouldn't run out of things to do. Kamara held out a beckoning finger, then leaned in and whispered a few suggestions.

Despite the rule of the double standard, things have loosened up. Nowadays, the traditional roles often reverse—some men are actually waiting for Ms. Right, while some good girls just want to get it on.

Bedroom News

Another secret sisters don't want to give up is that the sanctity of their bedrooms is a myth. In fact, the bedroom can be a source of effective strategies to be used later. Believe me, I've heard it all. That's why I know that good sex can make or break a relationship with a black woman. If a man can't do it right *and* fails to treat her right, he runs the risk that the next day all her girlfriends—and their girlfriends—will hear about it. Of course, fear of revelation is another pressure that keeps men locked into their protective John Shaft/spread-the-seed mode.

Celia made sure that every sister in her tiny suburb of Detroit, Michigan, knew that Lon, her Trinidadian ex-lover, was a "thirty-second mon." Celia was a slim, stunning young woman who modeled for local photographers when she wasn't temping as a computer software programmer. She met Lon at a church social and was captivated by his musical accent, perfect white teeth, and smooth dark-brown skin. Lon was a recent arrival in America and anxious to find a girlfriend. He was quiet and well mannered, and when they danced together, Celia was wowed by the way he "wound his waistline." Those swivel hips had to mean she was headed for a good time in bed.

A week later at Lon's apartment, Celia discovered that Lon's horizontal calypso was dazzling, but in a few seconds it was all over. Not long after, the phone rang, and Lon excused himself to take the call in privacy, in his living room. Celia listened by the door; it was obvious that Lon was speaking very affectionately to another woman. She dressed and left, and Lon never bothered to get off the phone to say good-bye. The next day, Celia had set off a chain of cell phone calls that alerted all the available females in the area that Lon didn't know how to handle a woman, in bed or out.

The Women's Secret Strategies

The Mission: Cheating

A woman usually cheats because she's got solid evidence that her man is unfaithful, or to pay him back for generally shoddy treatment.

Women hide their outside affairs far more successfully, but two wrongs never add up to a right. Negative behavior can only bring about negative outcomes. Whether the cheater is the man or the woman or both, no one wins at the cheating game.

Of course, some women cheat simply because they want to. Males and females are more alike than either gender wants to admit. Women are nearly as likely to do the dirty as men. Cheating women also employ similar strategies to cover their tracks. The difference is, women cover those tracks more efficiently. Unlike brothers, who tend to forget that loose lips sink ships, cheating women don't seem to need to brag about sexual conquests. Also, women have learned over the course of human history to make up for their lack of physical strength by working their feminine powers of beauty and cunning.

The strategies: hangin' with the home girls

Like the guys, cheating women enlist female friends to cover for them, and they work this tactic much more carefully, periodically checking in with each other to coordinate their stories in case the main man calls for his girlfriend.

Jasmine just knew her husband Desmond was cheating on her. Those mysterious absences without good reason, his overly suspicious attitude toward her—these were signs of his own faithlessness, but Jasmine couldn't prove it. When her car broke down one snowy evening, a fireman named John stopped to help. His caring attitude touched something deep inside Jasmine, and when he asked if he could see her again, she thought, "Why not? What do I owe my husband?"

Jasmine and John embarked on a torrid affair, thanks to the elaborate network of support Jasmine created with her girlfriends.

Jasmine had always been a social animal, and she made sure to cover up her dates with John by telling Desmond she was involved in a group project that involved good works among the less fortunate. She and her friends visited the homes of housebound old folk and overburdened single moms. That way, Desmond had no one place where he could check up on her whereabouts.

E-mail

Cell phones are a giveaway if the cheater answers a call from the wrong person. Cheating women don't need to talk; they just want to set up the next meet with the man on the side. Those tiny, portable e-mail machines are perfect for fleeting contact. So fellas, when a woman only gives out her e-mail, you've been warned that she's up to no good.

The day those portable e-mail machines came out, Sharon was at the store, handing over her credit card. Her long-term, live-in relationship with Albert wasn't working out the way she'd hoped, but Sharon wasn't about to drop him until she was sure that her new relationship with Rinaldo was on more solid ground. Meanwhile, she didn't even have to log on to her desktop and chance arousing Albert's suspicions. She kept her portable e-mail device in a tiny hidden compartment in her purse and simply used the bathroom as an excuse to check her messages.

The quickie

Forget the business trip—too dangerous. A few hours between the sheets at the local "don't tell" motel will do just fine. Most women have to balance the demands of home, children, family, and job, so they've learned to use their time efficiently. They don't need an entire evening or weekend to take care of business. Of course, some women occasionally allow themselves that indulgence if they can pull it off, but they are usually satisfied with an illicit hour or two.

Leticia actually preferred to keep her meetings with her outside man, Jerry, on the short but sweet tip. Those brief tastes kept him hungry for more, and since Jerry was married to her good friend Violet, quickies were less likely to arouse suspicions. Leticia felt a bit guilty about sleeping with her friend's man, but a girl's got to do what a girl's got to do. Besides, Leticia had never got over Violet's treachery when they were in high school and Violet seduced Leticia's steady boyfriend. True, it was a one-night stand at a party where the drinking had gotten out of hand, but Violet still owed Leticia this payback.

The wedding band protocols

Sisters don't want to bother with taking the band off and then possibly forgetting to put it back on. Besides, the wedding band clearly signals the rules of engagement: "You can have some, but don't even think about getting it all. I got a man who takes care of me." Ninety-nine times out of a hundred, the deal is just fine with the new man.

Sheronda still loved her husband, but he was chronically ill, and their lovemaking was infrequent and tepid. Ed suspected that his wife was getting her satisfaction elsewhere, but he understood and was grateful that she stuck with him and always came home.

Sheronda made it clear to her lovers that they were only passing fancies, and that her heart belonged to her husband. If a man tried to take it further, she blocked him at every turn. She didn't even want to be friends. She kept that area of her life separate from her home life by never giving out her telephone number and always seeing her men in a motel.

Just friends

Some men have a problem maintaining friendships with women, but, as Harry Belafonte once sang, "De woman is smarter." Women have the friendship strategy figured out—how to be "just friends" with a man. This is where it gets really baroque and slippery, because some women take advantage of their fabled ability to remain trustworthy and disciplined in their friendships with males. When a woman tells her man she is just friends with another brother, her man tends to believe it. Her man's trust then frees her to take the outside friendship further!

Janine took this ploy a notch higher by playing off her lover, Sidney, as a gay man. Sidney was one of those brothers with a hint of the feminine, but that pansexual vibe only made him more irresistible to the ladies. Sidney was all man, and a freak between the sheets who never tried a sex act he didn't like—but with women only. Janine, her man, and Sidney all moved within the same social circle, and Janine had been lusting for Sidney for quite some time when her man made a disparaging remark about Sidney's masculinity. That remark inspired Janine's ruse, so she played off her movie and dinner dates with Sidney as the equivalent of a night out with a "girlfriend."

It was me; so what?

Women don't bother with the *it wasn't me* ploy. Their tactic is infinitely more subtle and brilliant. Once they're caught out, some women readily admit to their guilt. Their genius is in insisting that their intentions were strictly noble. The cheating woman didn't intend to do anything wrong. She was keeping it honest and being faithful, but the male friend harbored bad intentions. He misunderstood the relationship and stepped out of bounds. If this strategy doesn't work, the cheating woman may go further and blame the affair on the husband's or steady partner's flirtations or past infidelities. She was merely taking righteous revenge. The beauty of this strategy is that the husband is left defenseless, and the cheating woman rarely has to resort to other defenses such as "It only happened once," or "I'm sorry, baby; it won't happen again."

Mona discovered that her husband was engaged in a long-standing affair, but she said nothing and acted as though everything was just fine. Mona went out and found her own squeeze, then put into place virtually every other strategy I've just laid out. She started out contacting her boyfriend by pay phone, then moved on to a cell phone, then to portable e-mail. She and her girlfriends came up with a youth talent organization that they used to throw off her hubby in case he called around to check her "I'm with my girls" story. Mona didn't even have to alert her friends to synchronize the story every time she was out cheating. Everyone knew the drill. No way would her husband get a story that differed from whatever Mona had told him. Mona's cheating game had moved from the satisfaction of revenge to an intriguing battle of wits. Mona and her friends were proud that their lying and cheating skills far exceeded the men's.

Yet Mona's marriage fell apart under the strain of isolation, cheating, and lies. When her husband finally figured out that Mona was cheating, her only response was "Yes, and . . . ?" Husband and wife had reached a stalemate where neither felt moved to justify, excuse, or apologize for their faithlessness. The children—who are often the smartest members of these families—picked up on the espionage game and were terribly hurt by the fallout from their parents' dysfunctional behavior. Everyone believed he or she was getting over, but they all suffered.

Brothers' Counterstrategies Against Cheating Women

The truth is that most men lack the patience and inclination for the intensely detailed detective work most women accomplish so zealously. Men who have reason to believe their women are unfaithful often go into shock. They can't believe their women had the audacity to do what they themselves do, and to hide it better. That state of shock usually weakens their brainpower, causing these men to react drastically. If the partner of a cheating woman does retain a degree of reason, he may put into effect any of the following counterstrategies:

Hire a private eye

Women sometimes hire private sleuths, but they are less likely than men to have the hundred dollars and up hourly fee. Since most men control the household money and are lazier, they are more likely to pay a detective to find out what is going on instead of asking a friend to help or snooping around themselves.

Erik didn't really care what his wife Joy did or who she did it with, but a man has to control his woman, and he didn't want word to get out that Joy was almost as active outside their marriage as he was. Erik liked to have his cake and eat it, too. He wanted to live the life of a carefree single man and at the same time come home to a home-cooked meal and a clean, comfortable apartment, thanks to the efforts of the little woman. And if he was horny, he would always have a willing sex partner waiting in his bed.

When his friends began coming to him with stories about spotting Joy riding around town in another man's car, Erik didn't waste any time confronting her. He simply thumbed through the Yellow Pages and hired a private eye. A week later, those rumors were confirmed. Joy was seeing another man. Erik threw her clothes out the window and changed the locks on the door while Joy was at work one day, then set about recruiting another shy, retiring female for the role of his live-in housekeeper-concubine.

Phone taps

Phone taps are a favorite male intelligence move. Women are adept at cross-referencing phone bills and credit card bills, but men love gadgets and playing spy. They'll buy up elaborate recording devices at the local spy store and set up a system to tape phone calls coming into the home.

Dennis did love Geraldine, and though he'd had several flings during the nine years they'd lived together, he genuinely wanted the relationship to continue. Since they'd had their daughter the year before, Geraldine was staying home, and hints from a nosy neighbor gave Dennis reason to believe that Geraldine was receiving a male visitor.

The thought of his woman in the arms of another man hurt Dennis deeply, but he had to admit he enjoyed comparison shopping for a hidden home recording system and then setting it up while Geraldine was visiting her mom with their daughter. Unfortunately, the second time Dennis checked the audiotape, he heard a steamy conversation between Geraldine and a man who was obviously her lover. Dennis was furious and sad, yet he had to admit that he also felt proud of his expertise as a spy.

The tunnel of love

Hard as it is to believe, some men try to determine whether their wives are cheating by sensing changes in the fit of their penis inside the wife's vagina. If the vagina seems larger than usual, he suspects someone with a larger penis is taking care of the husband's business. Other men become suspicious if the woman seems less interested in sex. Maybe someone else is keeping her satisfied. These are highly unreliable ways to determine whether a woman is cheating, yet a vagina's monologue can actually testify to faithlessness.

China actually was caught out this way. She was skilled at hiding her cheating, but her boyfriend, Adonis, was significantly bigger than her husband. In fact, during their love play, China once whipped out a measuring tape and discovered that Adonis was an inch wider and three inches longer. After repeated sex with her boyfriend, China's vagina actually had become deeper and wider to accommodate him. Her husband noticed the change and, with the help of a private detective, confirmed his suspicions. The husband confronted China and left her.

The Mission: Tricking a Brother into Commitment

Sometimes a woman believes she can't snare a man if she's honest about who she is and what she really wants, especially if she knows the man she's after isn't suitable. The man could be married or an obvious player, but she wants him anyway. So she presents herself in a way calculated to seduce him.

The strategies: the body double

This is a universal tactic employed both by men and women as a marketing strategy. The body double involves sending in a "representative" to handle the crucial beginning phase of a relationship. That representative is actually you, but it's a different and contrived version of you—a dog-and-pony show that presents you as someone you are not. Or you could concoct a more alluring and accommodating personality, a fantasy job, or even alter your physical appearance through weaves, sexy outfits, colored contact lenses—even bottom and front enhancers.

When Remi undressed at night, she didn't know whether to hop into bed or a bureau drawer. In fact, Remi at her day job was completely unrecognizable from Remi at the nightclub. All her life, Remi had been thin to skinny, so when miracle bras and booty-padded panties became available, she was thrilled at this easy way of enhancing her stick-straight shape. She boosted her new image as a sex goddess with a long, curly blond weave and startling blue contact lenses. The look was obviously false against her dark-brown skin, but the men she met didn't seem to mind. And Remi always insisted on keeping the lights off when they were in bed. She liked to move around a lot and focus on the man's pleasure. That way, he was less likely to realize that she didn't feel the way she looked.

Great sex

Some women fail to realize that the best way to impress and keep a man is through a pleasing personality, kindness, and attention. They believe that hot, no-holds-barred sex will get that dog and make him stay. This is especially true when a woman is after a committed or married man. The woman who wants him reasons that he's been getting the same old sex for years, even decades. The lure of new and different sex will dazzle and overwhelm him, and he'll leave the boring wife. The woman who aims to snare a married man through sex also engages in psychological seduction. She lies and flatters him shamelessly and convinces him that he's her sexual superman. Flattery is a very powerful tactic, but its power wears off. Even the power of sex eventually fades, so these women have to work fast to get over before the man wakes up to the reality that he's been manipulated through his ego and his loins.

Sonya let her friends know that she was the champion lover. She could make a man come on her demand or make him last as long as she wished. She had something special between her legs, and she used that asset to extract whatever she wanted from her love slaves. In fact, Sonya's skill as a lover and her vivid pretense at passion magnetized virtually every man she lured into her bed. As long as she was satisfied with money, gifts, and the knowledge that she was a mistress of seduction, everything was fine. But as her admiring girlfriends dropped out of the game to form more emotionally intimate bonds, Sonya began to want more from her relationships. The trouble was, she didn't have a clue about how to relate to a man as something more than a sex object to be conquered.

Withholding sex

Once a brother is totally addicted to hype sex, the seductress's follow-up tactic may be to withhold it. This strategy requires great skill. She has to know exactly when he's hooked, then dole out her sex infrequently, yet often enough so that sex becomes his reward for giving her what she wants.

Sonya loved to play this game whenever a lover balked at meeting her demands. Of course, she was never so obvious as to state that he had to pay if he wanted to play. She'd simply act hurt by his withholding behavior and suggest that she had to feel secure and loved in order to let go fully when making love. Sonya regretfully hinted that he needed to prove he cared, or, sadly, their affair would have to end.

Getting pregnant

When all else fails, some women resort to lock, load, and hold: they get pregnant, often without the man's consent. Some women will even tell the man that they use birth control when, in fact, they don't. Or the ruse can involve ensuring that sex is so sweet, the man lapses into temporary insanity and forgets to bag it. Some women even insist they are unable to get pregnant. The "tender trap" has snared many married and single men who had no intentions of sticking around. Of course, these men can't blame anyone but their own foolish selves.

Sally, a longtime member of the women's group, took pride in her ability to hunt down married men. Sally considered herself to be extremely independent, so married men fit nicely into her freewheeling lifestyle: she could keep company with several men at the same time and still be free to do her thing. Sally claimed that she didn't want any men to leave their wives, but she did have to expect their visits any time of the day or night. Of course, this entailed a lot of effort on her part. She had to maintain perfect grooming around the clock and visit the gym daily in order to maintain her shape. She also expended a great deal of mental energy on conning each man into believing that she loved him and only him. When she first joined my women's group, Sally had little insight into her attraction to married men. She had bought into her own "I'm too free for commitment" story. After a few weeks, she began to link her relationship pattern to her mother's sadness and frustration over never getting a man to commit. "Be it ever so terrible, there is no place like home." Sally slipped into the same pattern as her mother because it was familiar. Of course, Sally believed she was different from her mother because she didn't want commitment. She was determined to seduce, then abandon as many of these men as possible. Unlike her mother, she assumed a measure of control by putting together her own harem. Eventually, though, Sally fell in love with a married man and grew desperate to keep him. She took drastic action and became pregnant. His marriage did break up, but the man was so resentful over her trickery that he refused to marry Sally and became her reluctant, angry partner in raising the child.

Brothers' Counterstrategies Against Trappers

I'm the first to admit that a woman's feminine wiles and sexual heat can turn a strong man into a weak-kneed sucker. But brothers can avoid the tender trap with equally craven counterstrategies.

Condoms

Brothers are finally learning that the almighty latex is not just about protection from venereal disease. It's a safe-sex way to ensure that they're not caught out there with an "oops" baby. Some brothers even double-bag it to prevent accidents, while others actually refuse to have penis–vagina intercourse.

Hit it and quit it

This is a simple but harsh tactic: once the brother figures out what's really going on, he gets the sex, then jets before the woman can put her spell on him. Since love has nothing whatsoever to do with it, these men dispatch needy females with cold, calculating efficiency.

It's not mine: you're on your own

This is a simple but brutal defense: the man disavows all knowledge and responsibility of the pregnancy, especially if he believes he's been duped into fatherhood. He may insist on a paternity test, but even if it comes back positive, he'll refuse responsibility for the child. The result is court-enforced child support. The man might hide his financial assets to limit his liability, or just leave town and hide out. Even those men who accept their responsibility are often so resentful that they can take it out on their children.

Splitting: big head v. little head

This strategy has a long tradition among the brotherhood. Psychological splitting in this context occurs when the brother splits his personality into his sexual animal and his devoted family man. I call the first personality the penis or "Little Head." Little Head responds eagerly to the seductress, even if this woman is manipulating and devious. The second personality, or "Big Head," is the thinker. He wants to keep his family intact; no matter what tricks a woman pulls, no matter how good the sex, the brother remains "faithful," at least emotionally. The wife or steady girl is number one—the woman who rules his home front, takes care of the children, and has his back. The outside woman may get Little Head, but the wife or committed partner has Big Head. If the man ever gets confused and becomes tempted to exchange the old relationship for the thrilling new one, he relies on sensible Big Head to remind him of his priorities and tuck Little Head back in his pants.

Sonny thought he would school the other members of the men's group on how to divide one's attentions between a wife and outside women. No matter how many women Sonny had on the side, he made sure to be home for dinner on weekdays and by 2 A.M. on weekends. Sonny was a good father and provider. As long as he followed those rules, his wife was willing to look the other way. His women got Little Head, Sonny explained, but the wife had firm control of Big Head. Sonny boasted that his method ensured no single woman ever got complete control over him.

The Mission: Living off a Brother

Some brothers love sugar mamas, and some sisters crave sugar daddies. Society looks more kindly on arrangements in which the man supports the woman, but when a woman is with a man for his money, she's being equally mercenary and manipulative.

Strategies: no money, no honey

When money is her objective, a woman can pull out the full complement of feminine wiles, especially sex for barter. Women have used sex to keep men in line since Adam and Eve. The exchange might not involve cold, hard cash: If the man doesn't buy the dress or take her out for a fancy meal, she withholds services. If the man delivers what she wants, he gets sex. Professional mistresses lay out the rules of their game even more clearly: their men know that before they unzip their pants, they have to pull out the wallet. You could object that this behavior is a form of prostitution, but sisters counter that their strategy defends them from all the users out there.

Brothers' Counterstrategies

Hide the assets

Whenever the brother visits a mercenary lady, he makes sure to leave his good jewelry at home and thin out his wallet. He avoids discussing his finances or his work in her presence and deflects all her questions about his finances with vague answers. She never knows what he has, so she can't come after it.

Direct deposit

One fast-emerging tactic is to bypass the wallet altogether, where a paycheck can be examined or even removed by a mercenary babe, especially if he's susceptible to her charms. Some men play it safe by arranging for the job to make direct deposits into their bank accounts. This is their insurance policy against the women's attempts to tithe them for that 10 percent.

Secret job

A secret job on the side can take just several hours a week and put more money directly into the man's pocket, without the woman's ever finding out.

Renee complained loudly to the women's group about her difficulties in staying on top of her sugar daddy's finances. In the beginning of their relationship, she got as much money from Stanley as she wanted. They ate at the best restaurants; he bought her lavish gifts and often presented her with a check to cover her rent. Over time, though, Stanley grew wise to Renee. He knew he was being played, so he began hiding his assets. He worked as a salesman and claimed business was off, so Renee no longer knew how much money he earned. Actually, Stanley worked several jobs, but he kept two jobs secret. Of course, Stanley had already withdrawn his emotions from the relationship. Renee was focused on locating Stanley's money and squeezing as much as she could out of him, while Stanley was equally determined to get as much sex as he could without paying. All the energy they put into their cat-and-mouse game could have been channeled into developing true intimacy and a healthy relationship. The game finally played itself out, with no winners left standing.

The Case Against Strategies and Counterstrategies

We've had a bit of fun with these strategies and counterstrategies, but the results from all this gaming are far from funny. No matter how successful the strategy, how clever the intelligence gathering, or how devastating the counterstrategy, when trickery, dishonesty, and manipulation are the foundation of a relationship connection, the guaranteed result is disaster.

Secret tactics require focus, time, and energy that could be directed toward exploring more productive ways of relating to each other. One reason why we resort to strategizing is that too many of us go after inappropriate partners. Once you've chosen to pursue someone who's not right for you, you are far more likely to lapse into negative and manipulative behavior patterns to keep the doomed relationship going. We know that many of these negative choices and pointless behaviors stem from our crazy and dysfunctional PTSD. But knowing that our PTSD is behind much of this problem doesn't really help the situation, and all this strategizing is dead-end behavior that helps keep our PTSD going.

The only solution is to break this vicious cycle by refusing to behave in false and manipulative ways that destroy trust and create hate.

If you seek true romance and a healthy relationship, you don't need secret strategies, intelligence gathering, or counterstrategies. I'm not saying you have to show your entire hand as soon as you sit down to the game. Love should have an element of play, as well as mystery—especially when it's new. However, good relationships are not founded on games but on basically healthy and honest behaviors.

Are You Playing?

You don't need exercises, reality checks, and questionnaires to know whether or not you're engaging in strategies, intelligence gathering, or counterstrategies. Unlike many of our PTSD behaviors that are elusive to detect, you can spot a player a mile away.

While you read this chapter, you probably recognized some of your own behaviors reflected in the stories and patterns I described. We are all guilty of secret strategies to some extent at various points in our lives, even when we knew we were doing wrong. If you are still engaged in this type of behavior even though you know better, consider the following advice:

Stop blaming or taking revenge

There's no excuse—not even the bad behavior of others toward you—for manipulating other people, even for taking revenge. Take stock of how your own behaviors are creating manipulative, superficial relationships lacking in intimacy and trust.

Make a conscious choice

You have the power of choice: you can engage or not engage with someone who is manipulative. Once you know someone is engaged in war games, demand a cease-fire. Confront that person and ask for a more genuine style of interaction. Never lower your moral standards. If another person insists on playing games, confront him or her with the rules of fair play. If the person refuses to play fair, move on.

Never engage the enemy

If you know someone is not all he or she claims to be, or that this person can only offer a negative situation, don't walk away—run. If he or she belongs to someone else, don't even go there. If his or her first question is about the size of your wallet, move on. If he only wants to get into your pants and has no interest in your mind, turn away. Negative people often drop clues about their real motives during your first meeting. Allow your radar to pick up those clues so you don't need to take it any further.

Retire from the spy game

If you've been gathering intelligence and working secret strategies in order to maintain a long-term relationship, you're probably weary of it all. It's time to embrace the truth of your relationship pattern. If that truth hurts, ease the pain by fixing whatever is wrong. Work on developing healthier ways to relate with your partner, if possible. If the relationship is unfixable, end the war by moving on. Remember: negative energy yields negative consequences.

Maintain your dignity

Even if you believe you handle your games with craft, your behavior is underhanded and tacky. Again, if you are convinced you must behave this way in order to maintain your relationship, question that alliance. Trust me: this style of behavior and this relationship are beneath you.

Engage in reconnaissance missions

When you go out to meet new people, seek out those individuals who demonstrate healthy behaviors, so you stand a better chance of sharing a healthy romantic situation. Sincere people don't come on with patented lines or hit you with a directly sexual approach. They can even be shy and modest. Most of all, sincere people approach you as a potential friend.

A national children's magazine called *Highlights* regularly features the adventures of Goofus and Gallant, twin brothers with very different manners. Let's use that model to help you determine whether the man you just encountered is a Goofus or a Gallant, a man with potential for a long-term relationship. By the way, Goofus and Gallant have female counterparts.

- Say you're at a club. Goofus's approach might be to whisper in your ear, "You look good," as he grazes your shape with a wandering hand. On the other hand, Gallant introduces himself with a friendly smile and asks if you're having a good time.

- Say you're walking down the street. Goofus walks right up to you and asks, "Hey, baby, can I talk to you?" Gallant smiles as he passes by and says, "Hello." He leaves it up to you to smile back.
- Say you're at a party. Goofus is a complete stranger, but this is a *private* party, so he's not too shy to say he wants to take you home. Gallant starts a friendly conversation and, after a few minutes, offers to get you a drink.
- Goofus wants to know how many rooms are in your home, how much money you make, and what kind of car you drive, while Gallant enjoys discussing your common career goals and leisure pursuits.
- Goofus wants your telephone number but won't give you his. Why? Because Goofus is married or otherwise committed. Gallant offers you his work and home telephone numbers. He has nothing to hide, and he leaves it up to you to decide whether to give up your digits.
- Goofus wants to get into your pants; Gallant wants to get to know you.

You won't learn everything you need to know to weed out Goofus from Gallant men or women during your first meeting. These tips are designed to steer you toward people who seem open and sincere, and to head off game-playing manipulators. Once you are with someone because you truly want to be with him, and he feels the same, no one is pressured to engage in sneaky behavior to maintain control or get the upper hand. If you are not enough to attract that person to you, then the relationship is not meant to be. Do not resort to trickery to win him or her over; just move on.

Work Together

No one is perfect and no relationship is perfect, but it takes two dedicated people to make a relationship work. If a man and woman truly like each other and are interested in exploring the possibility of a long-term union, they should sit down together periodically and talk about making their relationship stronger. Each partner should never retreat to his or her side of the war zone in order to figure out how to outsmart the other.

Treat each other as equals

If we believe our partner is our equal, we do not have to resort to secret strategies or counterstrategies based on exploiting what we believe to be male or female weaknesses. If we respect each other, we treat each other as fellow human beings first. We no longer have to condemn our partners to a gender-based stereotype.

Play fair

Where there's genuine love and caring, there's no need to take advantage of someone financially or in other ways. There's no need to lie about who you are and what you want from the relationship. Love and exploitation cannot coexist.

Focus on the positive

If we focus on what's good and honest in all situations, our value system naturally opposes low-down behaviors such as secret strategies, intelligence gathering, and counterstrategies. We have a greater sense of who we are and of our purpose in life, which is to bring out the best in ourselves and in others. We've discussed how black men and women hold onto distrust and negative views of each other. Once we recognize that all this dysfunction is part of our

PTSD and that we're all victims of our history, we can become more compassionate and respectful and turn our attention to the goodness in our hearts.

Friendship first

Whether it's the beginning of a new relationship, a chance meeting, a serious dating situation, or marriage, your first goal should be to establish genuine friendship. Friendship creates the solid foundation of all relationships, including love and romance. If you are friends with your wife or partner, you do not need solace from someone outside the relationship. Your true friend is there for you, and your true friend does not wage war or spy on you. Your friend doesn't cheat or manipulate you or take advantage of you emotionally or financially. Of course, you must fulfill the qualities of true friendship yourself.

Every member in my Friday men's group and my Wednesday women's group has learned valuable lessons about the follies of secret strategies. At one point or another, some of them bragged about how they got over. Over time, though, new insights and the dismal results of their strategies forced each person to recognize that his or her behavior had been manipulative, negative, and self-destructive. Sure, the war stories were fun—even thrilling at times—but shame won out and motivated them to change their game plans.

Everyone came to realize that dysfunctional behavior saps time, energy, and love from relationships that should be nurtured. The games had prevented them from getting to know their partners deeply and establishing a level of intimacy that could have brought so much to both their lives. Everyone finally reached the ultimate conclusion that love—not scheming, defensive behaviors—conquers all.

CHAPTER SIX

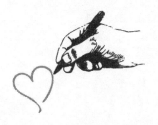

WE DON'T HAVE TO GO THERE: INTERRACIAL AND SAME-SEX RELATIONSHIPS

You may not know this, Dr. Jeff, but plenty so-called real broth-
ers—I'm talking about those buffed-up, thuggish types—are mak-
ing it with each other these days. They simply don't want to deal
with women's demands for commitment and emotional support. I
understand, though, because I've also found the love and caring I
need with my own. I never thought I could be that way, but my
older sister's friend proved that a woman could satisfy me sexually
and make me loved. My parents still don't know, and I haven't
even told some of my girlfriends. I plan to tell them soon, though,
because sisters need to know that they don't have to bang their heads
against a wall, trying to get brothers to treat us right.

I received this e-mail after a heated on-air debate about sisters who
find love with each other. This listener's words reflect a growing
trend among black women who say they are so fed up with the black
man's antics that they'd rather switch. Of course, some women are
truly gay and simply feel more comfortable about declaring their true
sexual orientation these days than they might have been in the past.
That's healthy. My concern is with those black women who are with
other women for the sole reason that they have bought 100 percent
into the prevailing pessimism about love with a black man.

I also endorse the truism that love has no color, but when sisters choose to date only white men or any other men but black men, that wholesale dismissal of black men is another major symptom of our PTSD.

Again, if you are a woman who's found fulfillment with another woman or with a man who isn't black, more power to you. It's also fine and dandy to test those waters in order to further your self-knowledge. But if your choice masks an attempt to escape from your problems with black men, you will never find satisfaction with anyone. Some women decide to reject all black men after too many traumatic relationships with brothers. These women invariably discover that their escape plan is flawed: either they feel trapped in their unhappy alternative relationship or they jump from one interracial or same-sex relationship to another. Why? Because they rushed into an alternative to black men without first considering whether or not that choice was right for them and without taking the time to work through whatever personal issues helped create their relationship problems. They're running from one accident site and moving on to create another disaster.

The same goes for some homosexual and bisexual black men and men who refuse to date black women if that choice is made out of fear and resentment. These men have bought into the stereotypical view of the dominant, angry, manipulating, demanding black woman or into any of the other stereotypes about black women. Again, homosexuality is natural for some men, and love knows no color, but defeatism can motivate a black man's choice to turn exclusively to his own gender or to women outside his race.

Bisexuality is a somewhat different story. My professional experience and my readings in current research indicate that many black men who engage in bisexual behavior are really gay, with only one foot out of the closet. On the other hand, the research indicates that many straight females who turn to other women are not innately gay—they seek out other women because they believe they can't receive emotional and physical satisfaction from men. These women are not embracing partners of the same gender as much as they are rejecting the opposite sex.

First, let's tackle the issues that might motivate a black person to date exclusively outside the race. In "The Beige and the Black," from *The New York Times Magazine*, August 16, 1998, writer Michael Linde reports that interracial marriages rose from a reported 51,000 in 1960 to 311,000 in 1997, and that the majority of these marriages were between whites and blacks. Blacks and whites coming together in this intimate way can be interpreted as a sign that racism in America is on the decline. But this development also reflects another manifestation of our ongoing PTSD.

I've heard too many black women state that they date white men because they know how to "treat a woman right." I've heard too many black men who refuse to date black women offer similar rationalizations. Yet these same black men and women are offended at the sight of other brothers and sisters with white or other nonblack partners. Sisters accuse black men who date exclusively outside the race of trying to get away with tired, triflin' behavior that wouldn't get by a black woman. They also accuse these men of playing off the John Shaft stereotype, as if their alleged sexual prowess earns them a free pass to behave any way they please. If the brother is successful, these women might accuse him of going outside the race to win a trophy partner that testifies to their superior status. Even if a brother hasn't achieved much in life, black women accuse him of believing that the white man's woman will elevate him on the social scale. As for brothers' opinions of sisters who date white men: these women are nothing more than stuck-up race traitors.

Again, I don't want to be misunderstood when it comes to the sensitive issue of race and sexual orientation. As a psychologist, I'm not concerned with the choices these people make. I'm concerned with the *reasons* for their choices. Falling in love has nothing to do with gender, race, ethnicity, or religion. Love of any human being is positive and healthy, and I have no problem with homosexuality, bisexuality, or interracial relationships. All love relationships are capable of mutual trust and nurturing as long as people aren't together because of a hidden agenda.

Joseph was living a lie. After many disastrous relationships with black women, he decided to date white women *only*. They were less angry and more intelligent than black women, he opined, and they seemed more receptive to him. Yet dating white women didn't make him happier. Joseph worried that he was losing his black identity; he felt like an Oreo: black on the outside, white on the inside. He sought out therapy to figure out what was going on. Did dating white women mean he was losing his blackness? As it turns out, dating white women exclusively caused Joseph to feel alienated from his true self and from his fellow blacks. He really wanted a woman who could understand him from the ground on up. He really didn't want to exclude sisters. A black woman would grasp more readily that so much of who he was today had been determined by his childhood in the rural deep South, and the difficult transition he'd been forced to make as a teenager when his family moved to Los Angeles. Now his social circle was made up exclusively of white women and their white male friends, so he was involved only in the concerns, interests, and issues particular to the white world. Joseph had believed that jumping into the white world would be the answer to his problems. Instead, it proved to be an isolating experience that made him feel like a stranger in the black and white world. After we explored this issue, Joseph accepted the observation that his relationships with both black and white women were conflicted and difficult because of his emotional issues. He began dating black and white women, which opened him up to both worlds.

Joseph was unhappy when he dated only white women, because limiting our relationships to the same sex or other races as a way to escape our relationship difficulties can contaminate other aspects of our lives. If this choice fails to deliver the happiness we seek, we can become truly depressed, because we sense something is wrong but we believe we've finally run out of options to remedy our situation. We believed the dramatic decision to change the sex or race of our partners would solve our problem, but when that choice fails, we are at a complete loss.

The experiences of people like Joseph, along with my instincts and experience, suggest to me that something is wrong with some current trends and that a significant number of black people engaged in alternative liaisons have leaped straight from disastrous opposite-sex relationships within the race into same-sex or nonblack relationships. They have not given themselves a break in order to work on their own relationship issues and prepare for the challenge of a healthier relationship with anyone. They have lost faith and taken what they believe is the "easy" way out. In other words, I believe that many of these alternative choices—whether interracial, bisexual, or homosexual—do not come from a genuine need to be with a specific person or gender, but from an attempt to avoid confronting the personal problems that created the negative relationship outcomes in the past.

Samantha came to therapy after a series of failed relationships with black men led her to date white men exclusively. Though Samantha stated quite defiantly that this would be her choice from now on, she also admitted that she was extremely unhappy because she was afraid to present these white men to her friends and family. She felt socially isolated; moreover, the switch hadn't really changed anything. After a few weeks, each white man she dated also began to withdraw from her.

She couldn't figure it out. Samantha worked hard—motor churning, gears turning, smoke coming out of her ears—to come up with some way for her ego to make it through these rejections intact. She told herself that the men lost interest because they were scared. Her drive highlighted their lack of direction in life, and dropping her was the easy way to combat their insecurities.

Yet Samantha tended to be overly controlling and suspicious, whether her partner was black or white. After a few months of therapy, she realized the problem wasn't one of race or culture. Samantha needed to work on how she behaved in her relationships or the fit would never be right, no matter what the race of her partner. If she wanted a real partner, she had to respect his choices. If she was really going to act like the strong woman she considered herself to be, Samantha needed to recognize that strength can also be defined as not knowing what you want, as long as you have the guts to admit it. She needed to recognize that strength was not necessarily speaking her mind at great, unsolicited length. Strength is also accepting rejection without having to put a flattering spin on it. When Samantha became truly comfortable with herself, she would no longer need to control how others perceived her.

Once Samantha was on her way to resolving her control problem—as well as the issues from her past that led her to keep picking the wrong men—she felt more comfortable about dating black men again.

Any behavioral choice made out of escapism or frustration never solves the problem. Avoiding our own issues also makes it easier to blame others for our dilemmas and to seek solutions outside ourselves, such as dating exclusively outside the race or seeking out partners of the same sex. On the other hand, withdrawing blame and taking responsibility for our issues offers the opportunity to resolve them and become more aware and fulfilled. When we fail to meet these challenges, we do not develop emotionally or spiritually.

My point is that you don't have to go there unless you are truly called! If you are in the closet, by all means, come out and look for a happy relationship. If you happen to fall in love with someone of another race, go for it. But if you suspect that you're making interracial or same-sex love choices because you've given up on your race or the opposite sex, take a good, long look at the possible issues within you that may have determined your choice.

Our behaviors are never the result of what "someone else did to me." We always have the choice to respond in any way to a situation: we can't shift the blame for our choices onto others. We take responsibility by withdrawing our stereotypical views, dismantling our anger, and acknowledging that our PTSD has damaged our relationships.

Now, let's track the origin in our history of the avoidance behavior I've termed "going there":

Going There

The Origins

We already discussed how our PTSD bred contempt for ourselves and each other and how we bought into the concept that we are inferior to white people. For hundreds of years, mixed-race folk—the fair-skinned and straight-haired among us—were our most sought-after romantic and marital partners. Of course, all this is rapidly changing with today's new appreciation of black beauty, but the psychosis lingers on in insidious ways. Many of us are still somewhat brainwashed to believe that whiter is better.

Many of us inherit color complexes from parents who gave us the message, directly or indirectly, that light is right, and who even pushed the brown-bag test to encourage their children to seek relationships that would "better" their lives and produce lighter, brighter grandkids. I must repeat: love knows no color, but many black people who refuse to date within the race suffer seriously from our PTSD because they've fallen prey to distorted and poisonous images about their own beauty.

In fact, I have no problem making the statement that anyone who dates exclusively outside the race suffers from a self-esteem problem. Our PTSD-related anger also plays a role in a black man's choice to be with a white woman, perhaps out of the need to get payback for slavery and racism. Some black men also believe white women are more compliant than demanding, intolerant and angry black women. On the other hand, some black women view white men as knights in shining armor who will save them from dead-end relationships with good-for-nothing, cheating, heartless, powerless-yet-posturing black men.

However, the current trend of turning to homosexuality or bisexuality in order to escape tackling our problems together is not rooted in the slavery of our past but in the thorny issues of our present-day dilemma. As the battle between our men and women heated up over the past several decades and homosexuality became more accepted, increasing numbers of us have found it easier to resort to this option.

In addition to our PTSD, many of us suffer from serious childhood trauma, and the resulting psychological issues can make us even more likely to give up on relationships with the opposite sex of our own race.

We each have our own sexual scripts that are influenced by everything from how we were held as babies, to the dynamic we observed between our parents, to our first sexual encounters. If we fail to resolve any issues arising from those experiences, we cannot be true to ourselves no matter whom we are with, because any relationship we create will be founded on all the wrong reasons—whether it's escapism or the drive to find a corrective emotional experience.

If we've experienced only dysfunctional relationships and all we heard from adults when we were children was that black men or women are "no good," that's all the information we have. We naturally act from that knowledge and come to view the opposite sex within our race as the enemy.

Brothers and Sisters Who Should Go There

Some brothers and sisters *should* engage in same-sex and even interracial love. For example, too many homosexual brothers are hiding in the closet and marrying straight women to keep their secret. One reason these men are stuck is that black society still tends to view homosexuality as an abomination. These gay men feel compelled to marry women as "beards," or even to deny their own sexuality to themselves. Of course, nature asserts itself sooner or later, so these men inevitably cheat on their wives with other men. How much better it would be for everyone involved if these men felt comfortable enough to live according to their true desires. Many black lesbians face similar pressure to find a partner of the opposite sex and deny their true desires in order to avoid censure from the community. Again, the best solution is to live according to your true self.

Some men who refuse to accept their true natures blame their rejection of women on "angry, confrontational, and combative females." These men claim tribulations with women drove them to seek solace in the arms of an understanding man, and that they are really bisexual. Again, many brothers who claim to be bisexual are also in denial. They are really homosexuals who use the perceived shortcomings of black women as an excuse for going there. Again, these men would be far better off—as would the women in their lives—if they simply accepted their homosexuality and stopped blaming black women.

Finally, for anyone who falls in love with a compatible person with whom he or she can create a satisfying, long-term relationship, race should never exclude that person simply because he or she is of a different race.

Those Who Should Not Go There

I've already mentioned that the growing incidence of black women's bisexuality is, in part, a glaring symptom of their dissatisfaction with brothers, and their widespread perception that the pool of available black men is all but dried up. Black men must bear a large share of the responsibility for the increasing incidence of bisexual black women. Our cheating, refusal to communicate and commit, domestic violence, and interracial relationships have turned many of our women away from us. Many black women are seeking out other women because they feel used and abused by men who believe the numbers game entitles them to bad behavior, including selfishness in bed. Many women who become involved in lesbian relationships report that only another woman takes enough time with foreplay. They accuse black men of rushing, refusing to experiment, and being selfish in bed.

If a woman switches for the right reason—love—she winds up a winner. Yet many sisters who turn to other women often become confused and uncomfortable and find themselves back where they started—yearning for a good heterosexual relationship. This is not emotionally healthy.

After a traumatic breakup with her fiancé, Anita completely

soured on men. Irene, a coworker, was a gorgeous lesbian and part-time clothing designer who seemed comfortable with her lifestyle choice and even exhibited a rare degree of personal freedom and confidence. Anita admired Irene's devil-may-care, fun-loving attitude and decided that lesbianism might be for her. She started going out with Irene and her lover to lesbian bars and eventually met Cora, an athletic banking executive. They began an affair. At first Anita was thrilled by the warmth and caring her woman lover showed her. They spent all their free time together, either alone or in the company of other gay women. One day Anita realized that her social circle had shrunk to a group of bisexual and lesbian women. Even when they went out on the town, she felt as if she was traveling through an alternate New York City, one that excluded all straight men. Though these friendships and her relationship were nurturing to some extent, Anita soon found herself pining for a heterosexual relationship. She couldn't figure out what was wrong. Women are supposed to be more loving, and Cora was more supportive than any lover Anita had ever known; yet Anita felt restless and unfulfilled. She sought out therapy and finally accepted that she really was heterosexual. What she needed to change was not the sex of her partners, but the type of men she chose and the ways in which she behaved within relationships. Once she realized that all her relationships had been vain attempts to get that corrective emotional experience, Anita felt ready to meet new men. Yet whenever she went out, she found herself at gay clubs or parties. She had limited her circle to settings that didn't involve straight men. The solution was simple. Anita needed to pick up the phone and reestablish friendships with the heterosexual friends she had neglected. Anita reintegrated herself into the heterosexual scene, but this time she was ready for an emotionally available man who was also open to building a relationship.

By turning to bisexuality or homosexuality or to partners of another race exclusively, we risk creating new destructive behaviors that will further entrench us in hate for one another. Those people we exclude from our dating or marriage pool become the reason for our unhappiness—the enemy. The people we reject in favor of partners of the same sex or a different race can even develop antipathy toward us.

Once we limit ourselves to partners of the same sex or other races, we tend to remove ourselves from the black community and restrict ourselves to the white world or the gay world. Many people who make this choice are surprised and dismayed by their sense of isolation from black friends and family.

Of course, if your alternative relationship is happy and satisfying, you will be less isolated, because when those who care for you realize that you are satisfied, they are naturally pleased for you and open to your partner. If your choice is based on escapism, though, you are more likely to be unhappy and become isolated from other loved ones because they sense that you are living a lie.

Again, if we choose any relationships out of a need to avoid personal issues, all that baggage from the past comes into the very same situation we expected to be our panacea. Relationships are relationships, and if we have unresolved issues, they will raise their ugly heads to disrupt any arrangement, whether it's heterosexual or homosexual, within the race or interracial. As Bob Marley once observed, "You can't run away from yourself." The best choice is to stay put and work it out.

Shirley was in a very abusive relationship of twenty years with her husband, Scott. He regularly berated her and beat her, and even put her in the hospital on several occasions. Shirley finally left her husband for the comfort and safety of her best girlfriend, Nadine. Neither woman had any previous experience with other women, but neither had ever known what it was like to be in a supportive relationship with a man. They had loved each other as friends for several years, so it wasn't difficult to allow that love to deepen into romance. Yet Shirley and Nadine soon began having similar problems. They couldn't understand what had happened to erode their bond, so they began counseling sessions with me. It seemed that Nadine had grown almost as verbally abusive and controlling of Shirley as Scott had been. Shirley admitted that she'd been involved in several other abusive relationships before her husband and Nadine—going all the way back to growing up under the thumb of her controlling and abusive father. Be it ever so terrible, there's no place like home. We tend to repeat whatever relationship patterns we learned in our childhood throughout our adult lives, or until we're finally able to resolve these primal emotional issues. Shirley naturally sought out abusive relationships because she was stuck in her childhood pattern and in finding that corrective emotional experience. How could she expect to establish a different relationship pattern with Nadine simply because Nadine was a woman?

After much therapy, Shirley began unraveling her pattern of abusive relationships. She realized she had leaped from one relationship to another, attempting to ease the pain over her abusive father with each partner: "This time, he'll love me the way Daddy failed to." The men in her relationships were stand-ins for the first man who rejected her—her father. Since each relationship failed to deliver the love she never received from that first man, Shirley incorrectly assumed that the problem was her choice of gender and that she would find the love she yearned for in a lesbian relationship. Shirley changed the sex of her partners, but she failed to change herself. Her unresolved issues reasserted themselves to create the same relationship dynamic with Nadine.

Shirley decided to address her issues in individual therapy. Armed with new insights into her choices, she began to pursue hetero-sexual relationships once again, this time leaving out the baggage of her past. Shirley and Nadine broke up, and Nadine also stayed in therapy to work out issues of control stemming from her own childhood.

Sammy felt he'd reached a dead end in his relationships. He had no idea what he could be doing wrong, so he figured after so many failed relationships with women, he might as well try men. After en-gaging in several unfulfilling homosexual relationships, he finally sought out therapy. He confessed to me that he received little physi-cal or emotional pleasure from these gay relationships, but he be-lieved that men could give him the love he couldn't get from women. Maybe another man would understand him better.

As therapy progressed, Sammy realized that all he'd been doing—with women and men alike—was trying to get that corrective emo-tional experience. His attempts to rewrite the script of his childhood with women never brought satisfaction, so he sought out men. Sammy didn't realize that he was recreating his relationship with his mother with each of his female partners, so he figured it was the women's fault. The real problem was that Sammy chose the wrong women—withholding types just like Mom—so each of these rela-tionships was doomed to failure. Of course, when Sammy sought out homosexual relationships, he naturally chose men with the same withholding personality because he was still seeking that corrective emotional experience. His relationship issues would never be re-solved until he could connect them to his primal experience with the mother who had abandoned him as a child and left him with rel-atives. Sammy wasn't even gay; he had sought out men as a last re-sort because he had no idea how to be happy in a relationship.

Sammy's unresolved issues with his mother created such difficulties in his relationships that he even made several suicide attempts. The confusion over his situation was driving him insane, he confided in me.

Sammy didn't know what love was or how to accept it. Even when a woman truly loved and wanted him, Sammy was unable to recognize it.

After several months of therapy, Sammy identified the issues with his mother that had been distorting his relationships both with men and women. He gracefully bowed out of his gay relationships and began dating women once again, this time choosing women who seemed more open and compassionate.

Whenever we engage in alternative relationships out of a need to avoid our issues with our race or the opposite sex, our self-esteem and our PTSD invariably worsen. We always sense deep down that our choice represents a self-betrayal on some level—that we're not acknowledging our real needs and taking care of ourselves by addressing them. But we don't know exactly what's wrong or what to do about it. Instead, we further doubt our identity and self-worth. We feel like a minority of one because we begin to lose the sense of where we belong and come to define ourselves as the odd man or woman out—both within our new social circle and our estranged community.

Interracial dating can be a thorny problem for younger people, especially black kids raised in predominantly white neighborhoods or attending predominantly white schools. Many of these black children become ashamed of their race or ethnicity because of subtle pressures to view the white lifestyle as mainstream and superior. When these kids experience discrimination or realize that they are viewed by others as black, despite these children's identification with white society, many of them become bitterly disappointed and hurt, especially if they are rejected by potential white dating partners. These black children grow up with a confused sense of identity and often lack the skills to interact with other black people.

Bjorn was a teenager with a white mother and black father who was raised in an all-white neighborhood. During those formative adolescent years, he wanted to do what all his white friends did— date white girls. There were hardly any black girls in his school and none in his neighborhood, so he wasn't interested in black girls. He had also been raised among his mother's white family, with little contact with his father's family, so he lacked a sense of his own physical beauty and the beauty of other people of color. All this set Bjorn up for a severe complex that made it even more difficult for him to approach white females. In addition, some of these girls' parents refused to let their daughters date a black boy. Bjorn was particularly wounded when he tried to pursue a relationship with Lauren, the red-haired, freckle-faced daughter of recent Irish immigrants. Lauren was just as sweet on Bjorn. The two got together most afternoons at the local library and often went out together with a group to the movies, the mall, or home parties on the weekends. But when Bjorn showed up alone one Saturday night to pick up Lauren for a date, that was the end of their little romance. Lauren's parents informed her the next day that she was not to consider Bjorn as a possible boyfriend. They understood that Bjorn was a fine boy, well raised by parents who, if anything, enjoyed a higher social status than Lauren's. They simply did not want their daughter dating outside their race or religion.

Bjorn was devastated. He didn't want to risk the same hurt with another white girl. His dilemma was tough. He wasn't attracted to black girls, and unlike his white male friends, he had problems getting dates with white girls. He lacked an identity as a black person, because his parents had raised him as a "mixed" child. All these issues took their toll. Bjorn's grades plummeted after he turned sixteen, and he began acting out his confusion and anger at school and in the home.

When his parents brought Bjorn to see me, we examined all these issues. One solution was to transfer Bjorn to a school with a mixed population of students who were black, white, and other races, so he could enjoy a more global view of his place in the world. His parents also decided to make more of an effort to introduce their son to black culture. These measures helped Bjorn feel better about himself and recognize the charms of both black and white girls.

Sometimes the best way to avoid a fight is simply to run the other way. But Bjorn's story and the other stories I just shared suggest that running away from our problems with each other will not end our war. Here are the key reasons we black people need to stick it out and work it through:

- Black men and women's only chance to overcome their mutual issues is through confronting them together. Escaping our problems through alternative relationships deepens our conflict and unhappiness. The same issues will continue to nag at us.
- Living a lie leads to unhappiness. We can never completely suppress our problems, no matter whom we choose to be with, because seeking answers outside ourselves means we are not working on changing the relationship style that gets us in trouble. Whether we're with a man, woman, black person, or someone of another race, the only route to a happier life is by taking a long look within and being scrupulously honest and true to ourselves.
- Most important, we owe it to ourselves as a people to stand on

the highest possible ground and become the best we can be, as individuals and as a community. The way to do this is by working together on resolving the personal and collective issues related to our PTSD. Escaping our problems through alternative relationships is merely the latest obstacle to our progress. We need to be clear about what we do and why we do it, in order to begin healing our relationships as black men and women.

Reality Checks to Eliminate Escapist Relationships

Our every behavior results from a self-statement we may or may not be aware that we've made. Authentic lives filled with authentic relationships require frequent reality checks to challenge the beliefs, stereotypes, and perceptions that can influence our choices and steer us wrong.

The Self-Statement Reality Check

This 10-step reality check exercise helps you identify any statements you may be feeding yourself that encourage and support your escapist relationship behavior:

Step 1: Identify and Write Down Your Self-Statements or Beliefs

- Black men are inferior to white men.
- Black women are inferior to white women.
- Black men do not treat black women well.
- White men know how to treat black women well.
- Black women are angry and confrontational.
- White women are compliant.

- As a man, only another man knows how I truly feel emotionally, spiritually, and sexually.
- As a woman, only another woman knows how I truly feel emotionally, spiritually, and sexually.
- As a man, the conflicts that erupt with sisters will not occur with white women (or other men).
- As a woman, the conflicts I have with men will not occur with other women (or white men).
- Men are abusive to women.
- Women try to control men.

Step 2

Read through the above statements. Do any of them "ring a bell," that is, describe your own beliefs?

Don't be afraid of the truth. You can handle the truth.

Step 3

Select each statement that describes your own belief. Write your own variation on its theme: For example: *As a black man, I won't experience the conflicts I have with sisters if I date or marry a white woman, because white women are more compliant.*

Step 4

Ask yourself, "Is this a fair statement?" Write down your response. For example: *The answer is easy. Such biased statements are never fair, especially if they are made out of anger, frustration, or disappointment.*

Step 5

Ask yourself, "Is this a generalized statement?" Write down your response. For example: *Again, the answer is easy. Statements that characterize a group in a general way are exaggerated and incorrect. Yes, some*

compliant white women are out there, but not all white women are com-
pliant, and some sisters are compliant as well. There are many instances
of brothers who had problems with a sister, divorced her to marry a white
woman, and wound up with even more problems.

Step 6

Discuss your statements with others to get the benefit of their
opinions, so you aren't limited to your own mind-set. If you open the
discussion to other people, you'll find that most rational folks refute
such sweeping statements.

Step 7

Expand your experience by observing how other people conduct
their relationships. Discuss with others the beliefs they hold about
relationships between men and women and within our race. Talk to
black married couples that seem to be relatively happy. Ask them
how they handle problems that come up. Explore how the real world
operates and discover that all people come in various dispositions.

Step 8

Write corrective statements to challenge your beliefs. For example: *Okay, I don't get along with black women, but they are not all bad.*
Maybe I should check what I'm bringing to the equation. Or: I am at-
tracted to white women, but not all of them are pushovers. Maybe I
should check out why I am more drawn to white women than to black
women.

Step 9

Read over your corrective statements as often as possible so they
can help you create more informed and conscious choices and actions.

Step 10

If you regularly challenge yourself with reality checks, your faulty belief systems will crumble and no longer create escapist relationship behaviors.

Here are additional action steps you can take to examine your relationship choices:

Work on Your Personal Issues

Take however long you need to unpack the baggage of your past in order to begin working out your personal and interpersonal issues before you become involved in any more relationships, traditional or alternative.

If the black men you chose were substandard or the black women were chronically angry, work on understanding why you didn't choose partners with the qualities you really desire. One individual never represents an entire race or gender. Interracial, gay, and bisexual love may be the fashion these days, but love does not follow the whims of fashion. Your choices should always result from your genuine needs and desires.

As I mentioned earlier, some of us choose partners of another race because our PTSD has created personal issues of self-hate and self-esteem. Those feelings can be so painful that we feel compelled—usually unconsciously—to project that negativity onto others, especially those people who remind us of ourselves. In short, it can be less painful to experience self-hate than to hate people of our race. The projection helps us avoid analyzing our antipathy and recognizing that it's really a reflection of our self-hate. Whenever we experience negative feelings about others, we should always ask whether our feelings and perceptions are influenced by problems with our own self-image. Whatever we judge as negative in others is usually nothing more than a mirror of how we perceive ourselves.

Here's a simple but effective exercise to help you combat the tendency to project:

Mirror Imaging

One day out of every week, question your perception of every single person you engage with, no matter what they say or do or how they appear to you. Try with all your might to determine if the qualities you dislike in that person reflect characteristics you suspect in yourself. Regular practice of this exercise will eventually give you the spontaneous and automatic habit of questioning all your judgments. This will help you determine whether you are really "getting" that person as he or she truly is or simply projecting onto that person your own feelings about yourself.

Building Better Relationships and a Stronger Race

If we want to improve our strength as a race and culture, we must dedicate ourselves to raising strong families united by strong values. Failing to spend time working on personal issues does not move us closer to this goal. Getting involved in alternative relationships out of a need to avoid the problems that disrupt our relationships with each other does not help us achieve this goal.

The ultimate winning strategy we need to follow is to become single-minded and dedicated to resolving our issues, to viewing each other as primary relationship options, and to tackling and working through our common issues.

If you have found a jewel of the same sex or another race, by all means, stay. But if you are unhappy in the alternative relationship you have formed out of your need to escape a negative behavior pattern or to avoid tackling your self-hate, examine other possible solutions that might bring you greater happiness.

If you suspect you have been dating exclusively outside your race or involved in gay relationships because you are fed up with the opposite sex and can't begin to envision a healthy relationship with a partner of the same race and opposite sex, try exploring the power of your imagination.

Imaging Your Relationship

Picture yourself in a beautiful relationship with a wonderful black person of the opposite sex. Frame this happy image in your mind. Allow your fantasies to explore the possibilities of the relationship. Make these fantasies your goal. Work toward realizing this goal every day, and soon you will believe in it so strongly that you can go out there and make it real.

In the end, love is always the answer. Love yourself, love your race, love your fellow human beings, and love your true sexuality, be it straight, gay, black, white, or other!

CHAPTER SEVEN

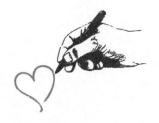

Healing War-Torn Relationships and Cooling Down Angry Partners

My man and I do nothing but fight. Everything I say, no matter how harmless, strikes him as wrong. He goes off, I go off, and all hell breaks loose. I don't know what to do. He's a good man, and I know he loves me. But we barely talk these days. This is killing us both, and I'm afraid we'll split up or kill each other. We have two small children, and I don't want them hurt.

These were the desperate words of a sister in my women's support group. Let's face it: when there's a problem in any relationship, you have only four options:

Change yourself.
Negotiate for change.
Leave the relationship.
Stay and be miserable.

This woman and her man—like too many other couples in our community—were locked so tightly into well-worn patterns of combat that neither was capable of seeing a way out. They were each incapable of hearing what the other actually said, let alone understanding what the other felt. They were stuck in what I call reactive mode, which means that their behavior toward each other was automatic, defensive, and explosive. Unfortunately, this rote, reactive type of anger can infiltrate almost every aspect of our relationships and human functioning.

Avenues of Anger

Let's examine the ways in which automatic and explosive anger has permeated our culture:

Language

From the youngest child to the most mature senior citizen, we use degrading terms to refer to each other:

- Bitches
- Ho's
- Niggahs
- Dogs
- Chicken Heads

These are just a few examples of the foul references that express overwhelmingly negative, disrespectful, hateful, and angry sentiments. In recent years, we've co-opted *niggah* and subverted its original racist intent. Today that term can be a badge of pride and a term of endearment, but *niggah* still bears traces of our unconscious self-hate and lack of self-esteem, and I question its widespread use.

Arts and Entertainment

When it comes to disrespect, we have to talk about music videos! Hip-hop videos are especially derogatory, with barely dressed women shakin' their booties to underscore the rhythm of a man's boasts about how many females he can sex whenever he wants. The women in these videos are reduced to mindless bimbos—decorative furniture with breasts, booties, and vaginas. Again, the vibe is hateful and disrespectful, and the message is that black men and women only cross the battle lines to make loveless sex.

Feature movies often expand on the music videos' demeaning intent. Even movies that seem like harmless fun, like "Friday," "Next Friday," or "How To Be a Player"—to name just three—base most of their jokes on the assumption that relationships between our men and women are, by nature, dysfunctional and full of anger.

I don't want to slam my fellow black authors, but too much black fiction these days is taken up with stories of black men and women employing underhanded strategies to get over on one another and then gloating about their misbehavior to their friends. Yes, some pulp fiction builds in a moral point about the need to cultivate greater self-esteem and mutual respect, but the anger, hate, and sneaky machinations are the main attraction, so that manipulation and dishonesty are elevated into strengths, and the dysfunctional behavior comes off like fun and games.

A newer generation of readers risks absorbing the weak value systems reflected in our entertainment and falling under the influence of these negative portrayals of black people and their relationships. The authors may use titillation to sell books, not to teach bad life lessons, but young readers will act out these negative scenarios in their real lives if more enlightened influences don't exert a greater influence.

Black People and Anger

We know that our explosive anger and animosity toward one another—as well as the secret strategies, intelligence gathering, and counterstrategies based on that anger—stem from our PTSD and our ongoing frustration over our underdog position in society. Fact is, we still lead in the following categories:

- Domestic violence
- Women abandoned while pregnant
- Single-parent homes
- Infidelity
- Children in foster care due to drug abuse or violence in the home
- Divorce

Anger and Conflict

All the research on marriage indicates that the number one predictor of separation and divorce is not disappointment with each other, financial problems, lack of sexual attraction, or falling out of love. The overwhelming cause of marriage failure in couples of any race is the inability to manage conflict. When a relationship is torn up by outbursts of uncontrolled anger, effective conflict management becomes impossible and that relationship hasn't got a chance. Anger and unresolved conflict are the major reason one of every two marriages today ends in divorce.

Even relationships between people who are merely dating are frequently plagued by conflict and anger these days. According to Sam Quick, a family life specialist at the Kentucky Cooperative Extension, physical and emotional violence contaminates an estimated one-fourth to one-half of all dating relationships.

Additionally burdened by the legacy of slavery, ongoing racism, and our PTSD behavior patterns, we black folk are not just lumped into these statistics about anger, conflict, and relationship failure—we lead them!

Again, our rage is a natural—even unavoidable—a consequence of our treatment in this country. But hate and anger can't be contained and directed exclusively at their real cause. These emotions spread and become so all-consuming that they can contaminate an entire life. Our anger, hate, and related self-esteem issues have trapped many of us in an ongoing process of implosion and explosion. That's why so many of our relationships are not merely troubled, they are time bombs—hazards to our psychological and physical health.

A study by researcher Janice Glaser measured the physical effects of a thirty-minute discussion of problems between marital partners over the following twenty-four hours. The more hostile the discussion, the more each partner's immune system was compromised throughout the rest of that day, that night, and the next day. Blood pressure elevated and stayed high for longer periods of time when couples demonstrated negative behaviors. This was not the case for couples that argued with less anger and more understanding.

The women in these couples seemed to suffer the effects of conflict more: they showed more immune system damage, making them more vulnerable to colds, heart disease, and cancer.

Temporary Relationship Insanity—TRI

We briefly talked about TRI in a previous chapter, but the topic is also relevant in this discussion. I have witnessed shocking displays of rage between men and women in my practice, on the air during my radio show, and when I've appeared on TV talk shows. It can get very ugly. I have worked with couples so enraged with each other that one or both threatened to end the relationship by ending the other partner's life. We're talking murder!

I'll never forget one couple on a talk show—both well-educated professionals—who had to be restrained by security. The wife was onstage first to tell her story. She wept copiously as she related how her husband had slept with her cousin and two other friends while she was pregnant with their first child. But when the husband took his turn and launched into a description of his wife's many infidelities, it was as if someone had pulled a rage switch. They lunged at each other like two mad dogs and had to be separated. No, this wasn't *Jerry Springer*. I won't reveal the name of the talk show, but it was one known for its elevated tone and the constructive approach of its host. Unbelievably, this couple was still sharing a home, although the husband was sleeping on the couch in the den. I stayed with this couple for two hours after the show was over, trying to negotiate a truce that would last long enough for the husband to enter the home and remove his belongings. Counseling was also imperative, and I arranged for them to start sessions with a psychologist in their area. But they were so locked in a pattern of rage that they needed to live apart for at least a few months to allow matters to cool down and then inspect the damage in order to determine if their relationship was worth saving.

You might be thinking, "Okay, Dr. Jeff, I understand why we are burdened with a legacy of rage that we've been handing down to each other since slavery, but these horrible things that lovers do to one another? They're plain insane. No excuses."

You have a point: that level of uncontrolled rage is dangerous, and it can't be excused. Still, we have to understand what's going on if we're ever going to find a solution.

What pumps up anger to the point where a relationship explodes and worse? I believe the cause is the automatic, unconscious, and negative way of reacting to a partner, called Temporary Relationship Insanity, or TRI. TRI is not just a black thing. TRI lives in all types of people, and it savages partnerships of all races every day.

TRI differs from anger in that TRI is fueled by such a mother lode of rage that it clouds all reason and can send the person in its grip spiraling into full-out craziness. Whenever TRI strikes, one or both affected partners lose all their perspective on reality. Once someone is caught up in the throes of TRI, he or she can become paranoid, delusional and truly insane. He or she views any behavior demonstrated by the other partner, no matter how innocent, as an attack that merits a counterattack. When both partners are lost in the madness of TRI, they lock into full combat. A dinner that wasn't prepared becomes a declaration of war: "She didn't cook because she wants me to starve!" Garbage that wasn't taken out is an attempt at enslavement: "He thinks he's better than me and he's trying to make me his slave!"

These examples are mild compared to constantly warring couples whose extreme rage leads to murder. Many domestic violence cases start with the husband isolating his wife from other social interactions. His paranoid, TRI style of thinking interprets any friendly exchange between his wife and another person as a deliberate attempt to disrespect him or as a threat to leave. He may become so enraged over the perceived betrayal that he'll beat her—even kill her. Love turning to murder is so commonplace these days that these horrific incidences of violence no longer merit front-page status. After all, stories of a man killing his former wife or current lover are a daily occurrence.

One graphic example of a TRI relationship that came to a bloody end is portrayed in the dark comedy *The War of the Roses*, a movie starring Michael Douglas and Kathleen Turner. After years of conflict and anger erode what was once a happy and peaceful marriage, TRI sets in. Loving partners turn into enemies, and their home becomes a war zone until it all ends with mutual murder. It's fascinating to observe how every behavior, whether innocent or not, is viewed by both sides as a threat that provokes yet another act of war. The film exaggerates to make its points and exploit the humor in this bizarre relationship, but the TRI of the Roses' marriage is not that far from the reality of noncelluloid couples.

Yes, TRI can take hold of any relationship, and it's always disheartening to witness love devolving into hate. But once again, black people are at greater risk for this extreme level of relationship dysfunction because of the anger that's built up in us over the centuries. Somehow, we find it easier to act out pain and rage over our history and the injustices of the present through warring with each other than to break down the rage and uncover its true causes. Our legacy of pain and anger has contaminated our relationships to the point where most of us now expect to be angered and disappointed by each other. We expect every relationship to end in war.

Let's break it down to discover exactly how our anger infiltrates our love:

Relationship Rage Catalysts

TRI is the thick, lethal stew of racial and personal rage that fuels our love wars. What conditions provoke TRI so that our troubled relationships explode into full-out war?

The conditions are many, but my clinical work and other professional experience suggest that the top issues that lead to relationship war include money, incompatibility, family or in-laws, and general stagnation of the relationship. Yet those issues mask even deeper causes for the kind of anger that tears relationships apart.

Nonspecific free-floating, or NSFF, anger

Nonspecific free-floating anger (NSFF) is generated in part by the daily stress of racism and its many inequities. As a result of racism, many of us experience what I call nonspecific or free-floating anger. There's no immediate or single reason for the anger that wells up toward the other partner, but the anger rises anyway. Many people refer to the welling up of this vague and chronic anger as "getting on my last nerve."

It's difficult to trace nonspecific, free-floating anger to a specific and immediate cause or causes, because NSFF anger can intrude itself anywhere among the details of day-to-day life, especially when a relationship is involved. Among dating singles, NSFF anger rears its ugly head in the form of hostile, suspicious exchanges when a man and woman meet for the first time, or similar behavior during the beginning phase of a relationship. NSFF anger is the reason why so many new relationships never get off the ground. The hostility associated with NSFF anger controls many of our psyches, so it naturally infects our relationships. Even when a relationship manages to get going, NSFF anger is guaranteed to cause trouble further down the line, as soon as someone's expectations for the relationship are not met. The result? More anger, and another relationship bites the dust.

Roberta began attending my women's counseling group because she felt completely incapable of finding a significant love interest. She complained that no matter how hard she tried she just couldn't meet someone. I asked why she believed she wasn't making that love connection. She thought about it for a moment and offered a possible reason. Perhaps she was too angry with men in general to make a relationship work.

Now that she looked back, she had to admit that every time she'd embarked on a relationship over the past few years, the man inevitably got on her last nerve. Gary, her last lover, was a quiet, patient man who'd really never given her cause for anger. He was always on time and considerate, and though he didn't exactly stoke her furnace to red-hot levels, he was a competent and considerate lover. Yet even Gary wore her out. By the time she handed him his walking papers, even the sound of his breathing as he sat next to her on the couch watching TV was driving her crazy.

We explored how this issue of anger played out and discovered that as soon as she met a potential partner, Roberta would be flooded with NSFF anger. We pursued the source of this anger until Roberta realized that her anger came from her preconceived notion that something had to be wrong with any guy she liked. After all, he was black, so he had to be a dog, just like all the other brothers out there. Angry behavior only elicits additional angry behavior. Roberta finally realized that the NSFF anger she brought to relationships was causing the men to respond the same way.

Carrie and Charles were together, but NSFF anger kept them from making that final commitment. They had been engaged for three years, but Carrie was frustrated because she still had no idea when they'd jump the broom. Charles was a stockbroker, and he pleaded that the volatile Wall Street market hadn't provided enough career stability to get married. He kept putting off the wedding date. When their arguments over the date turned verbally violent, they came to therapy. At one time, they'd seen most issues eye to eye; now they were stuck in NSFF anger, arguing over every little thing. They had gone down the slippery slope and landed in Temporary Relationship Insanity. Even the most insignificant, neutral word or act would be interpreted by Carrie as yet another trick Charles was using to avoid marriage. The final straw was when Carrie invited Charles to a college friend's wedding but Charles begged off. He had to finish financial reports and couldn't spare the time. From Carrie's point of view, Charles avoided the wedding because he didn't want to be reminded of weddings at all. Charles was able to clear up that misperception during our counseling session, but that wasn't a final solution. Carrie persisted in viewing his every behavior through the cloud of her TRI, and we couldn't spend our time analyzing and debunking every little misperception. The problem was that Carrie couldn't control her anger. She actually broke off the engagement several times, until they split up for good.

NSFF anger is most commonly seen in marriages or long-standing live-in relationships in which the day-to-day grind leads to relationship rut, or when new behaviors compromise the compatibility the couple once shared. Most often, though, the spouses are unaware of what's happening. They become irritated, as if they're getting on each other's nerves. Most of these relationships do not end in mutual murder, as with the Roses, but daily squabbles, petty backbiting, insult trading, and nagging recriminations are symptoms of the NSFF anger that makes relationships hell.

Charlene and Howard came to therapy for help with what they termed "communication issues." They had raised a fine family and were both consummate professionals. But twenty-five years together were beginning to take a toll on the marriage. They were civil to one another, but they'd stopped talking. Lack of empathy followed; then NSFF anger welled up over the gradual erosion of their relationship. The children were out of the house, and Howard had retired. He spent more time around the house now, puttering around with home repair projects and raising organic vegetables in his garden. Howard and Charlene had dreamed of this time in their lives, when their home would be quiet and peaceful and they no longer would have to meet the demands of their growing children. This was supposed to be their time, a golden period in which they could do whatever they wanted together.

Yet the more time this formerly loving couple spent together, the more distant they became. They had simply grown bored with one another, and romance had gone out of the relationship. Now they didn't even speak or touch. Both partners knew something was wrong, but neither knew what it was.

In this case, the problem was that neither of them had ever owned up to the resentments over small misunderstandings that had built up over time into chronic dissatisfaction. Taken on its own, none of these misunderstandings seemed important, but for each partner, the list of small grievances had added up to a pattern of self-ishness and thoughtlessness. Neither knew what to do about it, because it seemed silly to dredge up some minor incident from the past, so each withdrew from the other and retreated to his or her own emotional corner until the time came when they rarely stood on common ground.

Infidelity

Infidelity is a biggie, especially if the cheating is ongoing. Infidelity is the most combustible and destructive relationship issue of all. It's a giant betrayal, and when that betrayal is exposed, the wronged partner can react with explosive rage. His or her extreme level of anger is often expressed through vicious revenge behaviors, and it's not long before both parties are tearing at each other's throats. I have witnessed patients lose their marriages, children, and even their jobs over volcanic eruptions set off by infidelity.

Again, we can't forget that we as black people suffer from a habit of infidelity that is part of our PTSD, which means our relationships are plagued by more infidelity than others. The statistics you read in the Introduction bear this out. As a result, our relationships carry the burden of even more anger than those of other races. The betrayed partner can wreak revenge in many ways, and the relationship is often destroyed as a result.

Belinda's and Duane's parents urged their children to wait until they'd finished college and worked a few years before marrying, but Belinda and Duane had known they were meant for each other from the moment they set eyes on each other in Mrs. George's fifth-grade class. They married at eighteen, as soon as they were of age, and were deliriously happy to be alone together at last in their own little nest.

Neither had ever slept with another person, and neither felt any real desire for anyone but each other. Years went by, and the marriage prospered. Each partner supported each other's efforts to get a higher education, and Belinda won her bachelor's degree only one year after Duane. After six years together, they began to have a family and produced three adorable children—two girls and a boy—in five short years.

By now, they were in their late twenties and seemed to everyone who knew them to have the world by the tail. But Duane was getting restless. When the guys got together to "shoot the shit" and talk about females, he could only grin and nod, as if he understood what it was to play around and simply enjoy sex for fun. He wondered what it would be like to seduce a woman, to woo her into bed and then enjoy her different skin, different breasts, different sounds and smells.

Finally, Duane followed up on what began as a harmless flirtation with a regular customer at the job. After the first night he cheated, Duane was overwhelmed with guilt. He could barely look Belinda in the eye that night when he came home. But it was a little easier the second time, and by the fourth and fifth time, he had compartmentalized his affair, put it somewhere in his mind away from his marriage. He was just being a man, he told himself, and an outside sexual relationship had no bearing on his marriage.

Eventually, the inevitable happened: Duane got sloppy and dropped too many clues, and Belinda found out. She was devastated and took the children with her to live at her mother's for over a month. Eventually, she came home, but she couldn't get over the betrayal. After all, he wasn't the only one who'd wondered what it would be like to make love with someone else. But she had restrained her fantasies for the sake of their love and their marriage. A year later, Belinda decided to take up with another man. At first, she hid her affair, but something in her wanted to make sure Duane eventually found out. He knew he deserved it, but Duane was heartbroken and enraged. He was tormented by visions of his wife in this man's arms and couldn't bring himself to go near her. Even couples therapy couldn't help these two recover their former closeness. Two years later, Belinda and Duane were divorced. The following are some of the typical rageful TRI behaviors couples utilize to war:

Aggressive Behavior During the phase when the wronged partner suspects infidelity, or right after the infidelity is revealed, that person often responds with anger and aggression to the guilty party's every statement and behavior. This usually translates into much screaming back and forth. The relationship is constantly tense because any misperceived behavior, such as receiving a late-night phone call, or a letter addressed to the guilty party, becomes provocation for another explosion from the wronged party. The explosion can be verbal and even physical. When arguments erupt over subjects not related to the infidelity, the wrong party often throws that issue into the conflict.

Saleem and Trudy came to therapy because they were embroiled in one major argument after another. Saleem had cheated on Trudy two years ago. They had worked it out, allegedly, but it seemed as if Trudy still took every opportunity to throw her husband's past in his face. If he slammed the car door too forcefully, she somehow found a way to work in a remark about his former girlfriend. She had not recovered from the betrayal, and her aggressive behavior bore this out.

Passive-Aggressive Behavior Passive-aggressive behavior is less obvious, but it's just as painful to the recipient as overtly aggressive behavior. When a betrayed partner acts in a passive-aggressive manner, he expresses his anger indirectly. He does not say a word about the infidelity or even admit that anything he says or does is influenced by anger over the betrayal. When pressed, the betrayed partner insists that everything is okay and he doesn't need to talk about it. Yet dinners will be cold, clothes accidentally burned; the partner will be lifeless and nonresponsive in bed, or even refuse sex completely, stating that he is too tired or has a headache. All that rejecting behavior will be masked by a carefully cool and neutral attitude, and the wronged partner will never tie whatever he is doing to the partner's infidelity. Wronged partners will never even admit to hostile behavior. On the outside, they behave passively, but their actions speak just as aggressively as screaming, hurling plates, and even throwing punches. Because it's so sneaky, passive-aggressive behavior can be even crueler than directly aggressive behavior.

Ernie's affair lasted two years before his wife, Ellen, caught him red-handed when she spotted his car parked outside a room at the local "no tell" motel. Ellen was not one for loud scenes and throwing plates. She simply turned to ice. Ernie swore up and down that this was the first time he'd strayed, and he would break it off immediately. As far as Ellen could tell, Ernie was true to his word, but she couldn't forget what he'd done. She also couldn't unbend enough to tell her husband how much he'd hurt her.

Instead, Ellen resorted to more covert ways of expressing her anger and pain. Whenever they were out with friends, Ellen regaled the company with stories of Ernie's ineptness at home, even in bed. She always laughed when she recounted these tales at Ernie's expense, but everyone sensed the rancor behind them, and their friends stopped calling to get together. Whenever Ernie wanted to be intimate, Ellen found a convenient excuse—from a headache to an extra-lengthy menstrual period—and she didn't bother to make those excuses seem plausible. She was careful never to act overtly hostile so that Ernie could point to any particular behavior, but she made sure he suffered.

The Revenge Affair "I'm going to hurt you the way you hurt me" is the old reliable for wronged partners. Sometimes, the revenge affair kicks off immediately. In other instances, the wronged partner waits years to have the affair. Of course, two wrongs never make a right, and the level of anger that's packaged with a revenge infidelity only means that other people are being used, the main relationship is further damaged, and everyone suffers. In fact, this type of acting out can lead to murder.

I recently did a stint on a television talk show with several couples, each of which exhibited one of the infidelity behaviors I've just described. These were couples in which one or both of the partners had cheated, and one partner in each pair had come on the show to deliver an ultimatum. These couples were so angry at each other that they actually had to be kept in separate rooms before airtime, guarded by private security:

- Nancy had discovered that John had been sleeping with his ex-girlfriend for the past two years. Though he broke up the affair after he was found out, Nancy was not able to contain her anger over his betrayal. She made it her business to make his life miserable by yelling and screaming at John every chance she got. Her rage fueled her suspicions, so any innocent behavior, phone call, or errand became a clue that he had taken up the affair again. Nancy's aggressive behavior meant they were always embroiled in violent arguments.

- Joe knew for some time that his girlfriend Sugar was involved with her boss, yet Joe kept it all inside. He said nothing, but his passive exterior hid the fact that he was on a slow boil and threatening to bubble over. As a matter of fact, Joe's entire motive for appearing on the show was to finally confront Sugar about the affair. After everything came out into the open, Sugar revealed that the affair had ended long before. She'd sensed something was bothering Joe, because he was growing quieter at home, at the same time that he was becoming angrier and angrier over unrelated situations. He'd show up two hours late to take her shopping, or if she cooked him dinner, he'd eat only a small portion and leave the rest. An even stronger indication of Joe's passive-aggressive behavior was their dwindling sex life. Even when she did her best striptease, Joe would turn over and go to sleep. After confronting Sugar on the show, Joe admitted that his blood pressure had skyrocketed since he'd found out about the affair, and he was now on medication.

- A few months before the show, Lamont discovered that Celia was seeing his best friend on and off. Lamont confronted Celia over this several times. She said the affair was over, but he knew she secretly continued to date his friend every once in a while. Lamont was so angry that he found himself putting a significant dent in a bottle of vodka one night, then heading for Celia's best friend's house. They began an affair. Lamont had no feelings for Celia's friend, but it felt like the perfect revenge. He revealed the affair on air, but he still left the show feeling unfulfilled and extremely angry.

In fact, all the couples on that show left without any satisfaction. Their paybacks had failed to make them happy or resolve their issues. They eventually filed for divorce. But divorce is not the end for those and many other couples!

Divorce

Instead of solving the problem, the big "D" can actually further fuel relationship war. Divorced couples can remain tied to each other through ongoing anger and recriminations and, especially, through their children. Once a couple shares a child, their relationship is never over. Divorce can actually bring the worst out in relationships. Obviously, divorce is usually justified, but it doesn't have to be ugly. Divorce can result from a mutual decision to go separate ways, but most divorces are the end result of years, even decades of bitter fighting, anger, recrimination, and turmoil, and they're rarely pretty. These destructive behaviors often worsen during the process and even after the divorce, unless the ex-spouses purge their anger and move on with their lives. Of course, any unresolved problems from your first marriage will show up again in new relationships. Ultimately, the lesson from any divorce should be that we must learn to communicate and to love our partner in the way he or she needs to be loved—not in the way we want to be loved. Unfortunately, in some divorces, the anger becomes so overwhelming that the following weapons of war are the cruelest of all:

Assets Unless successful divorce mediation is achieved, there's little hope that the splitting couple can see past the haze of their TRI to make rational decisions about who gets what. TRI renders them incapable of realizing that they are only hurting themselves and their family, especially since protracted divorce battles usually siphon off joint assets into the attorneys' pockets. But warring spouses are often too involved in using money, children, and other assets as weapons to recognize their folly. I've even known some partners to be so enraged that they stopped working and lived in poverty rather than give up any money to the ex-spouse.

Mark actually sold his business for one dollar to his closest friend, then sold his loft apartment in downtown Manhattan for a nominal fee to his cousin and went back home to live with his mother—all to avoid paying alimony to his spouse and to keep the support payments for his children down to the bare minimum. Gail was just as determined to exact her pound of flesh from her ex. She hired a series of lawyers, who in turn contracted the services of several private detectives. After eleven years, when the children were actually teenagers, she was finally able to unravel the complicated trail of Mark's assets. Of course, the lawyers wound up with most of the money in their own pockets, and everyone had gone through eleven years of hell.

Children Children are often the weapons in ongoing battles between separated couples who share children. Usually the mother is struggling to get the father to become more involved in the children's lives, or the father wants to spend more time with his children.

One will complain about the other in front of the kids in an attempt to turn the children against the other parent. Most parents know better and are aware of the damage this behavior can do to a child's psychological well-being, but the parents do it anyway. They simply can't control the urge to commit character assassination on their former—or about to be former—spouse. In some cases, a parent will forbid the children to visit with or talk to the noncustodial parent, and the result is a scorching custody fight.

Child-support payments are another potential minefield for angry ex-spouses. The parent who pays support believes he or she is paying too much and that the child doesn't really see the money, or the parent who is supposed to pay support believes that withholding the money will hurt the custodial spouse. In reality, the children are the ones who are hurt. Whenever kids are trapped in the middle of a divorce, they are the biggest losers.

Raymond and Cherry's divorce became so riddled with attacks of anger and blame that they ignored the feelings of their teenage twin daughters and bashed one another in front of the children. Already confused by typical adolescent issues, the constant war between their parents pushed both girls over the edge. They began to act out sexually with boys. The judge officiating over the divorce ordered a psychological evaluation of the parents and the kids and determined that the parents were no longer fit to care for the children. The situation ended tragically with the girls taken away from both parents and placed with an aunt and uncle. Only two years after the divorce were the girls allowed to live with their mother and receive visits from their father.

Divorced Parents Are Not the Only Ones Involved in the War, Single Parents Are Raging Against Each Other Also. The single-parent home is yet another arena where our battles outdo those of our white and other-race counterparts. When people share children but do not share a home or marriage certificate, the anger is often fiercest. The mother may be raging because she feels abandoned by her baby's father after she's given him a baby—the ultimate gift. She may also be furious because the father does not spend enough time with the baby. For his part, the father may believe the baby was a ruse to trap him into a relationship, or the baby's mama is requesting that he spend time with the baby as her excuse to see him. Some dads even refuse to acknowledge the paternity of their babies and become resistant to both mother and child. Some moms actually lie about their children's true paternity.

Whatever the reasons for the parents' anger, these relationships between single parents can grow so heated that every encounter becomes an occasion for screaming, crying conflict. Children constantly exposed to ugly scenes between their parents grow up with warped notions of relationships, which lead them into the same negative patterns as adults.

I appeared as a guest on a talk show when the topic of the day was young men who believed they'd been trapped into a relationship through pregnancy. The young men were furious because they'd been forced to accept an unwanted responsibility and spend time with the mothers of their children. The mothers were angry and tearful over the men's lack of responsibility. The truth was probably somewhere in the middle. The women should not have attempted to trick young, irresponsible guys into relationships. At the same time, the guys were not really tricked into fathering babies. Some of these young men even tried to claim they'd been duped into having babies with the same girl three or four times! These couples fought so furiously that their babies received little attention and nurturing.

Once a partner or both partners believe that all weapons have failed to exact the proper amount of damage, they can turn to character assassination in front of family members, friends, and even workplace colleagues. The goal is to convince everyone who knows the couple that he or she is a victim of the evil partner or ex. Each partner is determined to destroy the other's reputation and portray him or herself as guilt-free—the innocent victim of the other partner's shoddy behavior and tactics.

Single, dating or married, no one is ever satisfied in these situations. The only way to bring about peace is to find ways to let go of our anger.

How to Heal Our Anger

Understand Where Your Anger Comes From

By now you know that the first step in resolving any relationship problem is to check our PTSD as a root cause. We've already seen how anger, even rage, is a natural consequence of slavery and racism. The rage we carry from our history feeds into our relationship anger, making it more likely to escalate into temporary relationship insanity, or TRI.

Once you understand the true source of your anger, you are better equipped to make a distinction between that old emotion and whatever is really going on in your relationship.

- Make a commitment to grow, both as an individual and a partner by taking responsibility for your choices.
- Keep in mind that whenever there's a winner and a loser in any relationship, both parties in the relationship actually lose. Work for a win-win situation.
- Respect and value yourself and your partner equally.
- Raise your children to be independent thinkers. Raise your children to be so aware that they can block out the Niagara of negative images and language perpetrated about us in popular music, videos, movies, and books. Work with your kids to help them understand that media messages should not dictate life. Teach them from the youngest possible age to respect one another and avoid obscene language and negative perceptions

about one another. Show your children by example that love and kindness are the highest ways in which human beings can relate to one another.

Okay, that sounds great, you may be thinking, but *how* do I start? How can I break out of my anger and change my relationships? Here's how:

Institute a Cease-Fire to Give You Cool-off Time

If your anger is contributing to the battles between you and your partner or potential partners, stop whatever you're doing. If you are cheating, stop. If you are wrangling over money and property, stop. If your arguments don't resolve issues and keep you locked in a vicious cycle, stop. If you are involved in a domestic violence situation, whether you're the perpetrator or the victim, stop.

If stopping means temporary or even permanent separation—sleeping at a cousin's house, checking into a hotel, or even going home to Mommy and Daddy—do it now. If you can't tell whether or not you are contributing to the anger in your relationship, seek an objective outside opinion—even consult a religious leader or professional counselor.

- Arrange peace talks as part of the cease-fire. These talks don't have to go on for hours. As a matter of fact, one long talk probably won't be productive, because you and your partner have forgotten how to discuss issues without winding up in violent arguments. Daily but brief discussions about the state of the relationship and the fact that healing must begin are often more useful.
- Peace talks and cease-fires should be immediate and ongoing

in order to better manage conflict and eliminate anger as consistently as possible. Once a major problem is squashed and resolved, keep talking anyway.

- Identify a time and special place where you can talk every day. Pick a time that works for the two of you, when you are both relaxed.
- Begin by defining exactly what is going on in the relationship. Talk about the major problems.
- Create "What's Going On?" questionnaires for each other. Write down your answers and discuss them. Take time to discover your true feelings, thoughts, and impressions. Think back to past actions you've taken to resolve issues, and see if they can be applied to the specific issue at hand. Think back to actions you took in the past that did not help. Avoid them.

  Here are some examples of questions or statements you can use:

  The specific issue I want to resolve is _____

  Three positive things we did in the past to resolve the issue are _____

  Three negative things that we did that we should not repeat are _____

  I feel _____ about our problems.

  In my opinion, these are our problems:_____

  In your opinion, what are our problems? _____
- Choose your battles carefully. Don't sweat the small stuff.
- Create statements that help answer questions about who, what, where, when, and how. The more specific you are about time, place, and specific behavior, the more open and accurate the communication. For example: "I want to talk to you about last Friday when we yelled at each other about_____"
- Stick to one specific issue at a time. Complaining all the time

or veering off subject to focus on nonrelated issues is counter-productive.

- Use "I" statements rather than "you" statements. For example, instead of saying *You* make me feel very hurt," try "*I* feel very hurt about what you said." "I want us to set up and follow a monthly budget," instead of "You always spend money recklessly."
- Don't play the blame game. Take responsibility as much as possible.
- Respect belt lines. Do not hit below the belt, that is, attack tender spots and personal vulnerabilities. That means avoiding such passive-aggressive statements as "You don't look so bad for a middle-aged woman."
- Institute a time-out rule. If one of you becomes angry and irrational, suggest a time-out in order to restore calm. Leave the volatile issue and come back to it later. Don't forget to come back to that issue. Never leave it unresolved so it can ignite another blazing battle.
- Go out of your way to put a positive spin on what you are experiencing from your partner. This places your intentions on higher ground. Instead of leaping to negative conclusions because of your temporary relationship insanity, create more generous interpretations of your partner's behavior. For example, if dinner is not ready, your first thought might be, "She was too busy cleaning the house or was too tired." When you get into the habit of going for the positive interpretation instead of the negative one, you will not only share a better relationship, you will also enjoy more peace of mind and a friendlier attitude and suffer from less anger.
- Before allowing your temporary relationship insanity to drive you crazy over a loaded word or behavior, ask your partner to explain what that word or behavior meant. On the other

hand, if you realize that your partner has misinterpreted your words or actions, explain your true intention. This maintains rationality and cuts off unwanted anger before it can build steam.

- No physical violence, ever.
- No name calling, ever.
- Keep the volume of your voice at a nonaggressive, nonthreatening level.
- Always stay in the here and now. Don't dredge up the past.
- No ultimatums, ever.
- No fighting in front of the children, ever.
- As part of each discussion, each partner should offer at least one compromise.

Thomas and Lawrence were a gay male couple referred to me because their last fight had landed them in court, where they were mandated to receive anger management classes and couples counseling. I immediately instituted a cease-fire, which was not very difficult since both men were very much aware that they faced possible incarceration if they were arrested for fighting again. I am proud to say that they followed every ground rule I've listed above and never again became involved in physical altercations.

How to Cultivate Calm

For some people, calming down means going into another room or taking a walk to the grocery store. For other folks, it's prayer, meditation, or yoga. For still others, it's playing hoops, reading a book, or watching TV for a while. Engage regularly in whatever activities keep you relaxed and stress-free, even if you don't feel angry at the time.

How to Address Your Own Temporary Relationship Insanity

This TRI reality check exercise enables you to play devil's advocate with yourself whenever you feel your anger rising, so you can calm down and maintain your reason.

Ask yourself the following questions:

- Am I really listening to what my partner is telling me?
- Is it possible that I am not really hearing his or her message and irrationally interpreting his or her behavior?
- Do I detect a consistently negative pattern in my thinking when it comes to interpreting my partner's words and deeds?
- Are there other, differing interpretations of my partner's words or behaviors from the ones I've made?
- Is there any rational reason why my partner would want to hurt me?
- Is my anger causing my mind to distort his or her words or behaviors so that I misinterpret them? This last point is extremely important. When we are extremely angry and caught up in temporary relationship insanity, we desperately need a reality check. If you can't get rational and calm enough to do this, call on a friend or another objective observer to help you get more in line with reality and understand what's really going on within the relationship. The difference is comparable to the Incredible Hulk's understanding of someone's words or behavior v. the interpretation of his calm and analytical scientist alter ego, Bruce Banner.

Eliminate Alcohol or Drug Abuse from Your Relationship

Alcohol and/or drugs turn an already combustible argument deadly. These chemicals further fuel temporary relationship insanity by deranging your already confused mental state. The consequences can be disastrous. Never argue while drunk or high, and if either or both partners have a drug or alcohol problem, address it right away or the situation will never improve. Chemicals never substitute for open communication.

Advice Tailored to Specific Groups

If you are dating:

If you are involved or have been involved in angry dating relationships, leave your expectations, past experiences, and anger at home whenever you go out to meet new people. That baggage from previous relationships won't help potential relationships get going. That baggage is what weighs you down and keeps you stuck in cyclical relationship patterns of explosiveness and failure.

Make an honest assessment of your anger and frustration level whenever you deal with a new partner. Analyze your opinion and respect level for the opposite sex. Your chronic anger with the opposite sex may cause you to interact automatically with potential partners as if they were mere stereotypes.

If you are a divorced or single parent:

Stop criticizing your ex-partner in front of the children. Separate your needs from those of your kids. Too often we intermesh our own needs and feelings with those of our children. For example, we may keep our kids away from our ex because we're convinced that it's better for the child. However, we're really separating the child from his other parent because we are too angry with our former partner to recognize our child's needs. A quick solution is to ask the child—if he or she is old enough to be verbal—whether he or she wants to see the other parent. If you consider that parent to be a psychological or physical threat to the child, make sure the visits are supervised. Of course, if the child has been molested by the other parent, then all bets are off and there should be no visits unless ordered and supervised by the court. In cases where the other partner does not want to take responsibility for the child, or a battle over visitation is ongoing, the parents should not engage in any contact. Your children will observe your anger and learn to behave in the same way. If you and the other parent cannot craft ground rules together on custody, financial needs and visitation in a calm manner, hire representatives to do this for you.

If you're a long-time spouse:

Those folks who have been together for a lengthy period of time and have lapsed into stagnant ways of coexisting can defuse the anger that results from boredom and increasing incompatibility by taking action to save their relationship. Many of the action steps and general suggestions I have already laid out will help. I also recommend attacking the anger and the early seeds of discontent by bringing back as much excitement and romance as possible:

- A kiss a day keeps the anger away. Try to have physical contact with your partner every day—if not a kiss, a touch or a hug.
- Sleep in the same bed every night with your partner, unless you are so alienated from each other that you need a cool-off period. But make sure not to do this for too long. Couples often initiate further estrangement by retreating to separate bedrooms.
- Get in the habit of addressing conflicts in your marriage as soon as they emerge. Never sit on the anger, allowing it to fester and grow.

- Make a commitment to deal with every issue that comes up.
- Keep romance alive with a quiet, romantic dinner out at least once a week. This curtails cabin fever that can lead to arguments or irritability. Also, when you're out among people, you tend to behave yourselves and argue less. Besides, an elegant, romantic dinner is relaxing and sensual.
- Always keep in mind that you are individuals with differences. Still, you need to set common goals both of you can pursue for the greater good of the marriage and family.
- Fornicate to avoid fighting. I give this advice to every couple. Marvin Gaye had it right: we all need sexual healing, and when couples stop making love, they stop communicating. The sexual energy they should be sharing converts into the negative energy of anger. On the other hand, your shared sexuality eases the daily strains of living and smooths out the wrinkles of marriage. Even if one or both partners are not in the mood, stick to a rule of making love at least once a week, twice a week, or even once a month. Do whatever it takes to get in the mood, whether it's a glass of wine, a warm bubble bath, sexy clothes, watching porno, or sex toys.

Genie and Roger had been married since the age of fifteen. By the time they were both thirty-five, they had been married twenty years. After Genie's breast was removed due to cancer, they were referred to my office. She and Roger wanted to discuss how the loss of her breast and the threat to her health could affect their lives and possibly alter their sexuality. They had a strong marriage, but the stress of these issues was a challenge. A few weeks before the surgery, they had found themselves beginning to act testily with one another. Despite the cancer, they continued their daily routines and responsibilities, but their sex life ground to a halt. After several sessions, they realized that one of their most effective stress reducers—not to mention favorite activities—was making love. Making love at least twice a week had kept their longtime marriage young and vibrant. We discussed how to return intimacy and sexuality to the relationship so they could recover their closeness and adapt to their evolving sexuality. The solution was simple: go back to making love twice a week.

Genie is now in remission, and Roger swears there's no difference in their lovemaking. Before the surgery, she slept in the nude, but now she wears a short T-shirt to bed, and Roger really enjoys the tease of a little bit of clothing.

We've talked a great deal in this chapter about how to manage our anger so that it doesn't destroy our relationships. I want to close this discussion by stating that anger isn't always negative. We don't have to be afraid of our anger, because that emotion is only a problem when it is not addressed, when it is allowed to grow unmanageable and destructive. Anger is a normal part of life, as well as an understandable legacy of slavery and racism. Anger can actually become a relationship ally if it alerts us to issues within that relationship. Anger lets us know that these issues need to be addressed and resolved so that relationship bonds can be strengthened and intimacy deepened.

If you are single and looking for the right person, remember that relationships can be worked on but never forced. You can avoid much heartache and trouble if you keep your eyes wide open and look for the following qualities in a mate:

- Commitment to personal growth
- Emotional openness
- Integrity

LOVE PRESCRIPTION

- Maturity and responsibility
- High self-esteem
- Positive attitude toward life
- Kindness and empathy
- Generosity

CHAPTER EIGHT

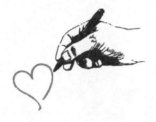

BREAKING THE CYCLE

We've learned that parents and other primary caretakers are our first teachers about love and that we've been passing down our distorted love lessons through generations of our children ever since our collective self-image was corrupted by slavery. Everything we've covered so far in this book underscores the point that, if we want to find genuine love within fulfilling relationships, we must first heal from the massive inferiority complex that resulted from being treated as less than human. We must drop the behavior patterns that once helped us to cope with our dilemma but no longer serve our best interests or the interests of generations to come. In the end, a community is only as strong as its parents.

As parents, we must find more positive and effective ways to advise our children, and more constructive behaviors to model for them so we can interrupt the legacy of destructive behaviors that are feeding our PTSD and destroying our community.

Let's take a look at the misguided messages we're giving to our children:

What Mama Says to Her Girls

"Never Trust a Black Man. All They Want Is What's Between Your Legs."

Whenever a young girl is bombarded continuously by this maternal message, she grows up into a distrustful, angry black woman who perceives all black men as manipulating, self-serving sex fiends. Black men don't stand a chance with a woman so walled in by automatic and universal distrust that she views every nice gesture or word as a bid for sex. Mama's "all they want is sex" belief creates paranoid women who defend themselves with a hostile or sarcastic attitude.

Either these women want nothing at all to do with men, or—if Mama advised her girls to "get them before they get you"—the daughters are mistrustful and rejecting.

Lisa came to therapy because she couldn't understand why she hadn't found a good man. She was a professional accountant, owned a beautiful brownstone in Brooklyn, and was very attractive and kind. Yet she was unlucky in love. Every time she became intimate with a man, the relationship crashed and burned. Lisa believed the only possible reason for these disasters was that these men were really only interested in sex and nothing more.

Her last relationship, with an electrician named Art, was the most disillusioning. Art was a hardworking man who juggled several jobs at the same time, doling out some of his work to other electricians so that he handled his business like a contractor. Art started work early and ending late, yet he always found time to appear at Lisa's doorstep, freshly washed and groomed, flowers in hand. Sure, he was often an hour or two late, but he always called to let her know he was delayed, and he never failed to show up.

Art was seriously courting Lisa, but Lisa couldn't handle those moments when she was waiting at home, watching the clock and fearing he was standing her up. Fantasies of Art at some bar, picking up on a young hottie and forgetting about her, crowded her brain. By the time Art arrived, she'd be so lost in those fantasies that her behavior took on an accusatory edge, even if she never voiced her suspicions. Art knew how much effort he'd put into making sure he saw Lisa regularly despite his busy schedule, and how much he'd reassured her of his deep interest in her as a longtime partner. He wanted a woman who'd greet him with a warm welcome, not a sarcastic, acrid tone of voice. Finally, Art backed off and left Lisa alone. Of course, Lisa simply figured she'd been right all along: he'd found someone cuter and younger because sex was all he had wanted in the first place.

A few weeks into therapy, Lisa began to consider the possibility that the problem was not that the men were after sex but that she *believed* that was all they wanted. Lisa's belief—not anything these men said or did—dictated her behavior with men.

Whenever Lisa became intimate with a man, she was fearful that he would abandon her, and unconsciously communicated her distrust by interpreting every neutral behavior as a rejection. This nice woman would turn into an angry, suspicious harridan, and the man would leave—Lisa's hostile behavior left him little choice. Upon further exploration, Lisa realized that the seeds of her distrust were planted by her mother, who had relentlessly drummed into her head phrases like "Never trust a black man; all they want is sex and the exit sign." Her mother's attitude had colored Lisa's perceptions. Once Lisa adopted a more open and healthy approach to men, her relationships improved.

"Get a Man with Money and Drain Him Dry, Sugar."

Daughters who grow up to this mercenary mantra develop a hoochy-mama approach. They don't even think about love; their trade is sex and money. When I was single, I dated some high-priced females with a price tag. You pay for the dinners. If you take them out to an event, you pay for the new dress. If you invite them to the apartment, you cater the food. They never dig into their own pockets, even to pay for a meal they cook in their own homes. Some will even stoop lower. The day of my wedding, an ex-girlfriend threatened to show up at the church and make a scene if I didn't buy her a television set. I didn't need the headache so I bought her the TV—a thirteen-inch brand X that communicated how little I thought she was worth!

We also can't ignore the fact that some black men reinforce mercenary female behavior. Pooty Tang clones rant, "Girl, I spent thirty-nine-ninety-five for dinner and a movie. I expect thirty-nine-ninety-five worth of booty tonight!" No wonder females up their price!

"You've Got to Do for Yourself; You Can't Depend on Them."

This spin-off from the "black men are lazy, no good, and only want one thing" advice turns young girls into overcompensating sisters who are convinced that if they don't take care of it *all*, their lives—and the lives of everyone around them will fall apart.

Many mamas who dish out this advice along with the breakfast grits are hurt, angry, and frustrated over their own abandonment by the fathers of their children. These mothers unwittingly ensure that their daughters will suffer the same pain, by teaching them to have low expectations of black men. Unfortunately, their advice is too often justified. Seventy percent of today's black children are raised by single parents—most often their mothers.

Lashunda came to couples counseling because she was fed up with her husband's unreliability. For his part, Clarence complained that shortly into their marriage he began suffering from feelings of worthlessness. Though Lashunda's take-charge attitude was "kind of sexy" while they were dating, he expected a more equitable arrangement after they were married. But Lashunda had a death grip on the reins of control. She refused to value his opinions on important decisions, and she said he wasn't even able to do household chores well enough to trust him to that job. She'd wind up kissing her teeth, shoving him out of the way, and doing it herself.

After Clarence injured his back and was put on a month-long sick leave, their life together became even more miserable. Lashunda was convinced that Clarence would never go back to work. She just knew she would have to carry the weight for the rest of their lives! Yet Clarence had never missed time from work before, never said he would stop working, and was back on the job after his sick leave was over.

Lashunda finally began to accept that she'd been brainwashed by her mother's barrage of warnings about "lazy black men" to the point where she couldn't give her husband the chance to be a fifty-fifty partner in their marriage. After that mental lightbulb switched on, Lashunda eased up and her marriage became happier than ever before.

"Black Men Can't Be Faithful."

This nugget of advice is passed on to daughters by mamas who've been bedded and abandoned too many times. Again, these ladies are not entirely wrong. We've already discussed the sad fact that black men are unfaithful to their marriages at a higher rate than men of other races and that this is, at least partially, a result of our PTSD. However, some black men are capable of fidelity to one woman.

One problem with this piece of Mama's advice is that the daughter may decide that since there's no hope of finding a faithful man, she may as well get involved with any man. She doesn't even bother to put forth the effort and patience it requires to find an honest man—the right man. The daughter never even thinks to demand fidelity as a requirement in her relationship. Of course, Mama's warning then becomes a self-fulfilling prophecy.

Joy, a member of my women's group, complained vehemently about the unfaithful men she'd dated. Gary, her last flame, worked at a record label where he met a lot of women, and he seemed to take special glee in stepping out with as many other women as possible. After she surprised him twice when she showed up at two concerts and caught him with a different woman at each one, she finally turned him loose. He carried on so fiercely about how much he loved her that she took him back, only to have him get drunk at a bar and try to pick up another woman right in front of her! That relationship and the others before it confirmed everything her mother, relatives, and other adult women had told her about the black man's cheating ways. Joy never considered the possibility that she had created this pattern of faithlessness herself, until other women in the group pointed out that Joy had chosen one faithless loser after another. Joy's low expectations and suspicious attitude even threw off her one good guy who tried in vain to prove his loyalty. Cheating men were so much part of Joy's life that she couldn't trust Glenn. If he so much as glanced at another woman, she'd be overcome with rage and tell him she knew what he was up to. Glenn, the honest guy, got her not-so-subtle message that cheating was expected, so he wound up cheating, too.

What Mama Tells Her Boys

"Your Daddy Ain't Shit!"

Abandoned by their men and forced to raise children alone, many mothers freely and frequently vent their anger and disappointment in front of their sons. Unfortunately, boys who hear "Your daddy is no good" or "Black men ain't shit" over and over, eventually interpret the message to include themselves. One: these boys grow up to believe that's what all black men are about. Two: these boys are almost men themselves. Three: these boys still yearn for the love of the absent or dysfunctional father, so the sons emulate the "no-good" behavior in an unconscious effort to win Dad's approval—even if he isn't around.

Yet many of these same single mothers also idolize their sons and give them a free pass on the very same shoddy behaviors they criticize in the absent fathers and "all black men." Mama winds up colluding with her son's wish to pattern himself after Dad by being lazy, irresponsible, and incompetent. The son grows up to fulfill Mama's negative observations about black men and is tortured by his conflicted relationship with his mother and all black women.

These boys are destroyed emotionally at a very early age and destined to act out their pain through destructive adult relationship behaviors.

Angelo was in his late teens when he and his mother came to my office for therapy. After pulling straight A's throughout grade school and high school, Angelo was now failing college. He'd also started using drugs and hanging out with the wrong crowd. His mom could not understand what had happened to her perfect boy.

The reason for Angelo's sudden shift in behavior became clear, though, when his mother compared Angelo to the father who had abandoned the family many years earlier. "I kept telling you how your father was no good," she screamed at her son at one point. "After everything I told you about your triflin' father, how could you turn around and act just like him?"

I interrupted her tirade to point out that years of hearing his mother bad-mouth his father had taken a toll on Angelo. His father was no longer in the picture, so all Angelo knew about his father—and what a man is about!—was whatever his mother told him. He had taken in all the negative statements she'd made about his father. Now Angelo had reached manhood, and he was acting out all he'd been taught about how a man is supposed to be. At the same time, Angelo needed to identify with his father, no matter how poor a role model his father was, and Angelo was naturally resentful over his mother's savage criticism of his father. As a young man, Angelo felt compelled to back up his father by molding himself in his image. Once Angelo and his mother were able to analyze exactly what was going on, the mother toned down her statements about Angelo's father, and Angelo understood that he could be his own man—a better one than his dad.

"Never Trust a Woman, Son. Your Mama Is the Only One You Can Trust."

We carry so much emotional baggage from our PTSD that our fathers don't trust other men and our mothers don't trust other women. Mamas pass on to their sons many negative images about their own gender by characterizing black women as conniving schemers who cannot be trusted, and in other negative ways. If Mama says this about her own gender, how can she be wrong?

These boys often grow up into women haters. Some also develop pathologically conflicted relationships with their mothers, in which they adore and hate her at the same time. (After all, Mama is a woman!) No other woman stands a chance with a mama's boy who may also live with Mama throughout his adult life. Even if he does marry, Mama inevitably intrudes herself into the relationship.

Harold was a good-looking fifty-year-old accountant who had never married. He turned to therapy because he just could not figure out why he'd suffered such a long string of bad luck with women— "nice girls who turned out to be jealous, evil bitches." He was attracted to each woman and had a good time in the beginning, but each woman's appeal always wore off after a few months. Harold would find more and more flaws and eventually lose interest. And he just could not figure out why these women were so unkind to his mother. These women were completely unfair, always trying to force him out of the home he'd shared with his mother since childhood. "Why can't they understand my devotion to the mother who raised me unselfishly, all by herself?" he asked me.

Of course, Harold needed to understand that the "flaws" he kept finding in each woman he dated could be traced to his mother's misguided message that "the only woman you can trust is your mama." Every time he'd brought a woman home to meet Mama, she found these women unacceptable. She was sneaky about her criticisms. When Harold called after these visits, Mama would ask subtle questions about the woman's clothes, her job, her past, and whatever else Mama believed would direct Harold's attention to the new woman's faults. Finally, Harold was able to catch on to Mama's game. He realized that no one but her would be perfect enough for her son. Slowly but surely, Harold is working on deprogramming his thinking so he can eventually create more balanced relationships. His bond with his mother remains intense but less pathologically so.

What Papa Says to His Daughters

"Watch Out for Those Brothers Out There!"

Many fathers echo Mama's warning that all men are lazy, unfaithful, untrustworthy, good-for-nothing dogs. How does Papa know this? He's simply confessing—and slyly boasting—about his past life as a dog. He knows how he got over on the ladies, so he bases his advice to his daughters on his very own bad behavior. These dads like to tell themselves that they only did what all young bucks do, but these fathers are actually unfairly projecting their own sins onto young men who could very well be innocent.

Of course, young women who receive these fatherly warnings grow up to become cynical women with little faith that they'll ever find a good man.

Jake's wife and daughter ordered him into therapy. This dad became simply unbearable whenever his daughter Jasmine had a visit from a male friend. She was a very respectable young lady who believed that her male suitors should spend time with her parents, but her dilemma proved the truth of the axiom that no good deed goes unpunished. Jake was convinced that every one of these boys was out to use and abuse his precious daughter, and he made no bones about his suspicions in front of her dates, who, naturally, couldn't wait to get out of his home and Jasmine's life. Jasmine and her mother were beside themselves. Jasmine began to keep her dates away from home instead of doing the right thing. Doing the right thing had brought her nothing but trouble.

Jake's paranoia resulted from his guilt over his own behavior as a young man, when his mission in life was to sleep with as many girls as possible. Once Jake understood that not all young men are like he was as a youth, he reeled himself in and realized how lucky he was to have a respectful daughter who brought boys home to meet the parents. Old habits die hard, though, and Jake still gives the boys a hard time, but not so hard that they're compelled to run.

"Be My Little Girl Forever."

This crippling message may not be delivered through actual words, but it comes across clearly through Daddy's actions. Smothering fathers inhibit the psychosexual development of their daughters by keeping them emotionally locked away in the attic of immaturity. The fathers are so afraid of what will happen to their daughters at the hands of men like themselves that they want their girls to remain virginal forever. Some dads even tell their girls directly that if they do date men, they are sluts.

These girls usually react in one of three ways. One: they obey and therefore fail to develop socially and emotionally. Two: they defy Dad but take in his perception of themselves as sluts and therefore suffer from low self-worth. Three, they become princesses with a Daddy's-little-girl mentality, who believe no man can measure up to Daddy. These women are in a constant search of the corrective emotional experience—a relationship that replays the emotional dynamic of the relationship with Daddy—but in the end, she gets to keep Daddy for herself, without the intruding presence of Mommy. Of course, no man will ever protect and prize her the way Daddy did, so these women wind up alone.

Carolina began to suspect that her relationships never seemed to work out because her perceptions of men were somehow off. She knew she had found some good men, but she could never settle for any of them. Her friends, cousins, and even her mother kept scolding her for letting good guys get away.

Therapy helped Carolina discover that no one was ever good enough because none of these men was Daddy, who had passed away many years before. When Carolina was a girl, Daddy was king and she was his princess. That relationship could never be recreated, so Carolina was trapped in the tower forever. The king was dead, but no other man had come along to take her out of the tower and place her next to him on the throne. Carolina admitted that her tendency to be self-centered caused her to write off the men in her life. Her therapy focused on learning what a genuine relationship between a man and a woman really is. Carolina came to understand that a relationship is about giving and sharing, not the worship of one partner. She began to assess the men in her life more realistically and stopped comparing her relationships to her experience with her father.

What Papa Tells His Boys

These same papas who smother daughters with their protection often turn around and dole out the opposite advice to their sons: "Be a player like Daddy," these fathers often counsel. Girls should be virgins, but boys should spread it around. The sons are encouraged to flirt with as many females as possible and rack up conquests so they can be viewed as real men. As I've already noted, even mamas can be guilty of handing out conflicting messages to their female and male children.

I've caught myself passing on a few "mackin'" messages to my seven-year-old son when I've asked him in public what he thought of a passing woman's looks. Yet, whenever my eight-year-old daughter talks about having a crush on a little boy, I become annoyed and worried. Thankfully, I recognized what I was doing and replaced my shameful behavior with lessons to my boy and my girl about friendship between the sexes and the importance of honesty and fidelity. If I had continued in my stupidity, as do too many daddies, my son would have learned from an early age that it is okay to act out behaviors based on the view of women as sex objects. My daughter would have grown up shackled by the double standard that still dominates today: men who date many women are ladies' men, but women who do the same are sluts.

What Mama and Papa Did

Of course, Mama and Papa can say anything they want, but they deliver their strongest messages through their actions. Actions always speak louder than words, especially to children, because they always look to their parents as role models and are heavily influenced by their parents' behavior. Psychological and sociological studies have proven over and over that almost everything we learn about relationships, dating, and love comes from the behavior we observed in our parents. It's not surprising, therefore, that studies also confirm that men and women in successful relationships tend to have been raised by parents in successful relationships. Sadly, homes riddled with domestic violence produce children who grow up to be either perpetrators or victims of domestic violence themselves. And if a spouse is unfaithful in a marriage, chances are his or her sons or daughters will grow up to be unfaithful or find unfaithful partners as well.

What about single-parent homes or homes where parents are coupled but have not made it legal? You can be pretty sure that unless parents take corrective measures to declare their bond before the world, the children will grow up to emulate those behavior models.

Ria brought her son and daughter to therapy because she was sick and tired of being abused by her children. She had been a battered wife, and the violence often took place in front of the kids. After many years, Ria finally threw out her abusive husband. The children had always been supportive of her and were clearly traumatized by what they had witnessed, yet as they grew older, they, too, began to be verbally abusive of their mother.

The kids were acting out their father's behavior whenever they became angry or frustrated with their mother, because they were falling into unconscious learned behaviors. Knowledge brings healing, and Ria's children used this insight to check themselves before acting out with their mother. Therapy also enabled these children to understand that their mother had been repeating with her children the same relationship patterns that had put her at physical and emotional risk with her husband. Though this family still goes through periods of instability, the abusive behaviors and patterns have stopped.

What Mama and Papa Should Do

If we want our kids to be in healthy romantic relationships when they grow up, we must model healthy romantic relationships as parents. We all have issues that affect our relationships. We don't have to model perfect relationships in order for our children to grow and find love. What is essential is to demonstrate to our children the willingness and ability to work on resolving issues in a healthy and constructive manner.

Keep in mind the following reasons why your children don't have to share your destiny:

Your Kids Don't Have to Imitate You

Those of you who are divorced, single parents, or never have been married don't have to fret that your kids are doomed to the same fate. Just put a little more effort into demonstrating to your kids that you are learning from past mistakes and moving forward toward a healthier relationship outlook and style. Linda was a single mother who was trying to work out her issues with relationships. Linda was attracted to bad boys, and her young son, Paul, grew up with a series of his mother's live-in lovers. He saw them come and go in pretty quick succession. This confused and disturbed the young boy, who naturally identified with these men. Finally, Paul expressed the fear to his mother that she would "get rid" of him if he misbehaved seriously enough. Fortunately, Linda had recently entered into therapy. She understood that she had to overcome her relationship problems and was able to reassure her son of her unconditional love. She also told him that her tumultuous love life was not the way it's supposed to be—that, in fact, she was not happy with this behavior pattern in herself and was doing her best to resolve it and find a more satisfying way to live.

Give Your Children Positive Messages About the Institution of Marriage

Even if you're not married, try to avoid passing on messages, attitudes, or behaviors that will make your kids cynical about marriage. Give them a greater chance to form their own healthy perceptions about potential partners and increase their prospects for enjoying successful relationships.

Sheila had been married and divorced twice, both times to manipulative and emotionally abusive men. Her first husband fathered Sheila's seventeen-year-old daughter, Ingrid. In therapy sessions with her mother, Ingrid described their living environment as extremely tense. Ingrid had loved her father, as well as her stepfather. However, she was not at all happy with how her father and stepfather had treated her mother. Her mother was also depressed, cynical, and angry about those relationships.

Ingrid and her mother were always close, and Ingrid had absorbed her mother's attitude about men to the point where Ingrid's own relationships with her father and stepfather suffered. She barely saw her father and refused to communicate at all with her stepdad.

Sheila decided both of them could use therapy. During the sessions, Sheila began exploring how she had infected her daughter with her negative views of her husbands and of men in general. Ingrid was her mother's confidante and friend, and Sheila freely verbalized her anger at men, often condemned marriage as a losing proposition, and generally portrayed herself as a victim. Once Sheila assumed her share of the responsibility for her unhappy relationships and dropped her victim role, she began to feel better about men and her future relationship prospects. Her new attitude freed Ingrid to address her own concerns and issues in therapy and change her own perceptions for the better. Ingrid's relationships with her dads improved, as did her relationships with boys. Sheila is now in a long-term relationship, and Ingrid is happily married with two sons.

Stop the Violence

If you and your partner argue violently or you've sunk into domestic violence, seek an intervention. Work it out in therapy. If necessary, get out of the relationship. If you don't stop, your kids will mimic your behavior and engage in the same destructive relation patterns as adults. Healthy is as healthy does!

Taquanda called my office in tears. Her seven-year-old son and eleven-year-old daughter had recently started to abuse her verbally at home and in public, calling her "reject," "jerk," and other choice epithets. Finally, her son, Sekou, punched Taquanda in the stomach during an argument. Sekou was also hitting girls in his class and was suspended from school pending a psychological evaluation. Taquanda was beside herself. She could not figure out what she was doing wrong as a mother. She was kind to her children and always disciplined them in a nonphysical and appropriate manner. I invited her, her husband, and the kids to a family session. Dad didn't show, but the rest of the family came in. The kids were upset and confused. They said they did not know why they were so angry with Mom, that they really loved her and thought she was a great person. The truth soon came out. It also explained why Dad did not show up.

Domestic violence was a daily occurrence in the home, with Dad verbally and physically abusing Mom in front of the kids. Whenever the children became frustrated, they simply emulated behavior they'd modeled from their parents, even though they had no particular agenda of their own with their mother. Since Dad refused to get counseling alone or with the family, therapy focused on helping Taquanda get out of the relationship, at least temporarily. Once the father left the home, the kids' aggressive behavior subsided greatly.

Through the course of this family's therapy, I also learned that both Taquanda and her husband had been raised in homes scarred by drinking and domestic violence. If Taquanda had not sought out help, that family legacy would have continued indefinitely, down through the generations.

Don't Bad-mouth Your Children's Mother or Father

If you bad-mouth your son's father or your daughter's mother, your child will naturally believe your criticism also applies to them, because children always identify with the parent of the same sex. On the other hand, if you bad-mouth your son's mother or your daughter's father, the child will come to believe that all people of the opposite gender are "no good." Either way, your child's prospects for a good relationship are compromised.

Suzanne's ex-husband, Robbie, had been a terrible husband, and now that they were divorced, he wasn't performing much better when it came to sending his minimal support payments and taking his son for overnight visits. Suzanne was struggling to support herself and her son, as well as attend graduate school, and she couldn't help expressing her frustration over Robbie's irresponsibility in front of her son. Her son never objected; how could he? His mother was justified, but he couldn't help feeling guilty, as if he were the cause of his mother's distress, especially since he was a male, just like his dad. In fact, Suzanne's constant harping about her ex eventually created a boomerang effect. As her son grew older and left the home, he tended to seek out his father, whom he'd missed so much when he was younger. Except for duty calls to keep the peace, he avoided the company of his mother because she was still obsessed with "that no-good father of yours."

Hire a Mental Cop

As parents and adults, we need to install a "good cop" in our minds. That cop has to be on alert, nonstop, checking whatever we say or do in front of our kids and blowing the whistle whenever we get out of hand. Tell your cop to use all the insights and tools for change you've received from this book. Let that cop keep you under constant surveillance to help you short-circuit negative behavior and substitute more positive behavior as soon as possible. Not only will your relationships become happier and more satisfying, but you will also become a better role model for your children.

Martina, who worked in computer programming, decided to give herself a silent "cancel, cancel" message every time she caught herself saying or about to say something negative and nonconstructive in front of her four children. At first, she tended to hit the "cancel" button after the offending remark had already slipped out. As time went by, she learned to actually stop a thought in its tracks, before it even had a chance to express itself aloud. Soon, she discovered she was automatically thinking in a more positive and constructive way.

Yes, this process requires work, but this is not the time to throw up your hands and grumble about how much work you already have. If we swallow our pound of cure, our children will need only the ounce of prevention we give them as loving, caring parents.

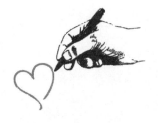

CONCLUSION:
FILLING YOUR LOVE
PRESCRIPTION

So what's the bottom line here? We've tracked all the ways in which our PTSD and the destructive behaviors it has created have put us at odds with one another. Now it's time to get busy and banish the specter of Mr. Charley.

He may be the master of our disaster, but only we can clear away the mess of the generational and reactive behaviors that decimate our relationships and weaken our individual and collective mental and physical health.

Loving connections are key to our survival as a race. Uprooting hundreds of years of negative experiences and behaviors requires work, dedication, soul-searching, and the courage to take responsibility for our individual beliefs and actions.

Once we are able to give up the ghost, we will reap the benefits of our work and consider ourselves in a new and more generous light. Our self-esteem will rise. Our interactions will become more authentic, respectful, and loving.

We all better understand the importance of loving relationships since September 11, 2001, when terrorist attacks exploded our lives in America. Americans slipped into a state of shock. We were outraged at the violation of our borders and the callous acts that took thousands of innocent lives and left countless family members and friends in deep grief. That mourning continues to cast a pall over our nation, for the remains of husbands, sons, daughters, relatives, and friends are still missing, perhaps never to be found, and our sense of safety is lost.

Incredibly, out of this horrible tragedy, positive changes are under way. Our nation and its people have come together in a spirit of co-operation never witnessed before during our lifetimes. That new spirit of unity and consideration has even changed our personal relationships, as singles and as couples. Behavior within marriage and on the dating scene has humanized, and we are beginning to acknowledge that love is really what matters.

In speaking to friends and colleagues and, in particular, observing and talking to my clients "on the couch," I have learned that since America was confronted with its vulnerability and mortality, life in the singles and dating world—as well as relations between married couples—has taken on a whole new significance.

Sex is no longer enough. Those marginal relationships where folks got together just to knock boots or get their batteries recharged are falling by the wayside. Now that our lives have taken on a new meaning, trivial relationships for sex, with little to no emotional involvement, are going kaput. Today's dating goal is to establish a permanent and stable relationship. In these dark days, people want more. Sex is always great, but we also need someone who can offer comfort, stability, and solace.

As I write these words, I am still receiving a rash of calls from men and women who are caught up in major reassessments of their lives set off by the September 11 tragedy. They are wondering whether their sexual dalliances were nothing more than silly diversions from their true life paths—to pursue healthier relationships that offer love and the opportunity for personal growth alongside another human being. I've even received several calls from guys who are upset, even slipping into clinical depression, because they can no longer get a boost from their old reliable habit of "hitting it and quitting it." All that seems empty and meaningless these days, but they don't know what else to do.

Then there are those longtime couples who have been on the fence, awaiting the "right" time to get engaged or married. Perhaps they were waiting for that salary promotion, or a better job, or that professional degree. All of a sudden, now that we've witnessed so graphically how our lives can be snuffed out in an instant, waiting for that ideal moment doesn't seem like such a good strategy.

The ideal moment may not happen for the next few years or more. Now that our nation has launched what is sure to be a long, costly, and dangerous war against an enemy that has secreted itself virtually everywhere on the globe, we're beginning to realize that time is not on our side. The time to bond is now, and that may be why many couples who were putting off their unions are getting engaged and setting the dates. As one engaged couple told me in therapy, "We are ready to march into our uncertain future together. We don't want the clock running out on us."

On the advent of World War II, Fred Astaire sang to Ginger Rogers, "There may be teardrops ahead, but while there's music and laughter and love and romance, let's play the music and dance!" Or as Prince put it more succinctly, "I'm going to party like it's nineteen ninety-nine!" He was only three years off.

Those songs seem to reflect the sentiments of many young singles following the terrorist attacks. While we are still able, while we are still alive, let's go out—to the bars, the clubs, and house parties. Let's go out with old friends; let's meet new friends. Let's dance, talk with each other, and enjoy and cherish each other's company, because now, more than ever, tomorrow is promised to no one.

In a weekly group I conduct every Tuesday for singles, one member after another has been discussing how they have been attending one party after another. They explain that they now possess a *joie de vivre* they never felt before. They want to live life fully and enjoy every moment possible. One member, an obsessive-compulsive who was terrified of contracting HIV despite practicing safe sex to the point of celibacy, reported that the harsh realities of September 11 brought him to his senses. He realized that his fears of disease were unrealistic and exaggerated, and that he could have sexual relationships and still be safe.

When the horrific events of September 11 unfolded before our eyes, we all realized that if ever there was a time to be bonded with a significant other, this is the time. Even strangers supported each other and clung to each other, especially right here in big, bad New York City, where singles were reputed in the past to treat each other like disposable objects. One couple after another has been telling me how glad they are to be married and have a partner during one of the most difficult periods in our history. Other couples that I work with, who had grown apart and emotionally estranged or who had become bored with the sameness of marriage, began undergoing breakthroughs and discovering reasons to rekindle their love and their relationships.

As chaos took hold in the aftermath of September 11, husbands and wives turned to each other for support, strength, and guidance. Many married brothers who had previously complained loudly and frequently about the old ball and chain now confess how much they look forward at the end of each day to coming home to the wife and kids—their shelter from the storm.

Marriages that had taken on the cold and airless void of outer space, in which neither partner heard the other's screams, began warming up. Spouses who had stopped communicating verbally, emotionally, and spiritually began talking to each other and offering each other comfort.

My own wife began calling me several times a day, just to say she loves me. Instead of being impatient at the interruption and turning off my cell phone, I welcome her warmth. I need this contact with her more than ever.

Many brothers I'd been treating for their chronic infidelity were overtaken by a powerful urge to put more focus and commitment into their effort to reprioritize their personal lives, to give up the girls on the side and work harder on being faithful in their marriages. Sure, they may slip up and fall off the wagon, but at least they're trying harder. Three or four of these clients even quit their running around, cold turkey. Their "aha" realization that these affairs were trivial, silly boosts to their egos made the change easy. Who can blame them? If an enemy were to drop a bomb on us, I'd rather spend my last moments at home with my family than in some stranger's bed.

On the downside, I have also received calls from more than one couple in need of crisis counseling because they'd been planning to have their first child but, after September 11, were unsure about bringing children into a world of bio-warfare and possible nuclear war.

My advice to these prospective parents was to carry on with their lives and build their families. We can't allow terrorists to compromise our futures.

Our renewed sense of the importance of love is the silver lining in the dark cloud that now hangs over us. Our instinct for survival has been awoken and, along with it, a greater appreciation of what we mean to each other. Whether single, committed, or married, we are all more aware and mature people today than we were on September 10.

We now realize that mutual respect and love are our sustenance; they will keep us strong during the days of uncertainty ahead.

The apocalyptic beginning of this new century offers us the opportunity to reclaim a sense of normalcy despite this crazy world. I hope and pray that we will not forget the valuable lessons on the importance of love and relationships taught to us by September 11. We can survive, but we can only do so if we acknowledge our need for each other.

I began this book long before September 11, by describing myself as a correspondent-analyst in the war between black men and women, but I didn't tell you why I cast myself in this role. Even before the events connected to that trauma, I had observed that virtually every problem my clients presented—men, women, and children—could be traced to the deterioration of relationships between our men and women.

The war against terrorism may be long, but it will end. Our future as a race—and as human beings—depends on ending the less obvious but very real war between the sexes. The peace effort begins with you. Whenever you work on yourself, you're in concert with countless others who are striving to become more realized, more loving individuals. What we need—what the world needs—now more than ever, is love, sweet love.

LOVE PRESCRIPTION

Ending the War Between Black
Men and Women

Jeffrey Gardere, Ph.D.

About this Guide

The suggested questions are intended to enhance your
group's reading of LOVE PRESCRIPTION.

DISCUSSION QUESTIONS

1. What are the symptoms of Post-Traumatic Slavery Disorder? Is it a real disorder or just an excuse for bad behavior?

2. How has Post-Traumatic Slavery Disorder created conflict between black men and women?

3. How does Complacency-Denial Syndrome keep people stuck in relationship ruts?

4. Why is blame fueling the war between black men and women? What are the payoffs for playing the blame game?

5. How have black people internalized negative stereotypes about themselves, and how does that affect their relationships?

6. How do black people themselves keep negative self-stereotypes alive?

7. What are your secret strategies and counterintelligence?

8. When is it not healthy to go *there*—that is, form interracial and same-sex romantic relationships?

9. What are the most effective ways to cool down anger and heal our relationships?

10. How can we prepare our children to form healthy, fulfilling romantic relationships throughout their lives?

INDEX

Index